THE HERBAL LEXICON

THE HERBAL LEXICON
In 10 Languages

Kate Koutrouboussis

AEON

First published in 2019 by
Aeon Books Ltd
12 New College Parade
Finchley Road
London NW3 5EP

British Library Cataloguing in Publication Data

A C.I.P. for this book is available from the British Library

ISBN-13: 978-1-91159-795-7

Typeset by Medlar Publishing Solutions Pvt Ltd, India

www.aeonbooks.co.uk

*Dedicated to Christopher Hedley who inspired, to Panos
for motivation and to my parents Pietro and Rozsi*

CONTENTS

PART I
THE HERBAL LEXICON

PART II
THE INDEXES

ACKNOWLEDGEMENTS

Lina Stenemo; Marco Anganaro; Józef Godlewski from Herbapol, Poland; Beata Palfalvy, St Steven University, Hungary; Cailleau Herboristerie, France; George Sfikas, Dimitris Loupis; Faruk Tuncay; A. Minardi & Figli, Italy, for help with herbal identification and to Panos, Natalie, Alexandra, Diana and Titi for translating 'How to use the Lexicon'. I am very grateful to all for the help they gave me.

Kate Koutrouboussis was born and brought up in London by an Italian father and a Hungarian mother. She acquired a number of further languages by extensive travel, and by marrying a Greek, and after taking a course in Herbal Medicine in London she saw an opportunity to combine her interests in languages and plants. She lives in Greece.

How to use the Lexicon

If you are an English speaker and want to know the Hungarian word for Shepherd's Purse, turn to the English index in Part Two and find Shepherd's Purse. Beside it you will find a number, in this case 137.

Next, go to number 137 in Part One and below the Latin name *Capsella bursa* and listed beside **H** you will see Pásztortáska, which is the Hungarian name for Shepherd's purse. If you know only the botanical name go to Part One where the plants are listed alphabetically under their Latin names and below will be the name of the plant in the various languages.

E = English; **F** = French; **G** = German; **S** = Swedish; **Sp** = Spanish;
I = Italian; **Gr** = Greek; **H** = Hungarian; **P** = Polish; **T** = Turkish

The same system applies to any of the other languages in this Lexicon. The purpose of this book is to help the herbal traveller, from students to professional biologists in the field, herbal retailers and wholesalers, people living away from their own country and medical herbalists. I have mainly kept to herbs which grow in Europe and the Mediterranean but have included some from the rest of the world which are commonly used in Europe.

I anticipate that this Herbal Lexicon will be very useful, not only for Europe and the Mediterranean but for Asia, Australia, and the Americas.

Comment utiliser le Lexique

Si vous êtes un locuteur francais, desirant connaitre le mot hongrois pour Bourse-à-pasteur, allez dans l'index français partie 2 et cherchez Bourse-à-pasteur. A côté vous trouverez un numero, dans le cas actuel le numero 137, ensuite vous allez au numero 137 dans la partie 1 puis sous la definition latin *Capsella bursa*, et à coté de la symbole **H**, vous trouverez le mot Pásztortáska, qui est le nom en hongrois pour Bourse-à-pasteur. Si vous connaissez seulement le mot botanique, alors allez directement dans la partie 1 ou les plantes sont listées alphabetiquement sous leur nom en latin et en dessous vous trouverez le nom commun de cette plante dans la langue recherchée.

E = Anglais; **F** = Français; **G** = Allemand; **S** = Suédois; **Sp** = Espagnol;
I = Italien; **Gr** = Grecque; **H** = Hongrois; **P** = Polonais; **T** = Turc

Le hongrois n'est qu'un exemple. Le même système s'applique à toutes les autres langues de ce Lexique. Le but de ce dictionnaire est d'aider le voyageur botanique, les etudiants, les biologistes professionnels, les herboristes, les marchands d'herbes medicinales, ou les personnes voulant connaitre l' equivalent en vocabulaire des herbes de leur propre pays.

Je me suis interessée principalement aux herbes qui poussent en Europe et autour de la méditerranée, mais j'ai rajoute celles qui sont connues dans le monde entier et fréquemment utilisées en Europe.

Pour conclure, je pense que ce dictionnaire botanique d'herbes sera très utile, non seulement pour les Européens mais aussi pour les habitants d'Asie, des Etats Unis ou de l'Australie.

Gebrauchsanleitung

Deutschsprachige, die das ungarische Wort für Hirtentäschel wissen möchten schlagen das deutsche Inhaltsverzeichnis im Teil 2 auf. Dort finden sie Hirtentäschel und daneben eine Nummer, in diesem Falle 137. Im Teil I steht unter der Nummer 137 die lateinische Bezeichnung *Capsella bursa* und unter H werden Sie Pásztortáska, die ungarischen Bezeichnung für Hirtentäschel finden. Wer nur die botanische Bezeichnung kennt, sollte im ersten Teil suchen. Dort sind die Pflanzen nach ihrem lateinischen Namen alphabetisch angeordnet und darunter die Pflanzennamen in den verschiedenen Sprachen.

E – Englisch; **F** – Französisch; **G** – Deutsch; **S** – Schwedisch; **Sp** – Spanisch; **I** – Italienisch; **Gr** – Griechisch; **H** – Ungarisch; **P** – Polnisch; **T** – Türkisch

Ungarisch wurde als Beispiel verwendet, das gleiche Prinzip gilt aber auch für alle anderen Sprachen.

Dieses Buch soll eine Hilfe für den botanisch interessierten Reisenden sein.

Es richtet sich an Studenten und Botaniker und Biologen, Gewürzhändler und Grosseinkäufer, Leute, die vorübergehend in einem andern Land wohnen und Spezialisten für medizinische Kräuter. Es werden hauptsächlich Kräuter, die in Europa wachsen, aufgeführt, aber auch einige aus andern Kontinenten, die in Europa bekannt sind und verwendet werden.

Zum Schluss möchte ich sagen, dass ich glaube, dass dieses Kräuterlexikon nicht nur für Interessierte aus Europa und den Mittelmeerraum nützlich sein wird sondern auch für Interessierte aus Asien, Australien und Amerika.

Så här använder du lexikonet

O m du är en svensk högtalare och vill veta det ungerska ordet för Lomme, vänd dig till det svenska indexet i del två och hitta Lomme. Utöver det hittar du ett nummer, i det här fallet 137. Därefter går du till nummer 137 i del ett och under latinska namnet Capsella bursa och listat bredvid H så kommer du att se Pásztortáska som är det ungerska namnet på Lomme. Om du bara vet, går det botaniska namnet till del ett där plantorna listas alfabetiskt under deras latinska namn och nedan kommer det att vara plantans namn på de olika språken.

E – engelska; F – franska; G – German; S – svenska; Sp – spanska; Jag – italienska Gr – grekiska; H – Ungerska; P – Polska; T – turkiska.

Ungarn är bara ett exempel. Samma system gäller för något av de andra språken i det här lexikonet.

Syftet med denna bok är att hjälpa växtbaserade resenärer. Från studenter till professionella biologer inom fältet, växtbaserade detaljhandlare och grossister, människor som bor ifrån sitt eget land och medicinska herbalister. Jag har huvudsakligen hållit på örter som växer i Europa och Medelhavet men har inkluderat några från resten av världen som vanligtvis används i Europa.

I slutändan anser jag att denna växtbaserade lexikonet kommer att vara mycket användbar, inte bara för Europa och Medelhavet, utan för Asien, Australien och Amerika.

Cómo usar el Léxico

Si usted es hispanohablante y desea conocer la palabra húngara para Bolsa de Pastor, consulte el índice español en la Parte Dos y encuentre Bolsa de Pastor. Junto a él encontrarás un número, en este caso 137. Luego, ve al número 137 en la Parte Uno y debajo del nombre latino *Capsella Bursa* y en la lista junto a **H** verás Pásztortáska, que es el nombre húngaro para Bolsa de Pastor. Si solo conoce el nombre botánico, vaya a la Parte Uno, donde las plantas se enumeran alfabéticamente bajo sus nombres en latín y a continuación se encuentra el nombre de la planta en varios idiomas.

E – Inglés; **F** – Francés; **G** – Alemán; **S** – Sueco; **Sp** – Español; **I** – Italiano; **Gr** – Griego; **H** – Húngaro; **P** – Polaco; **T** – Turco.

El húngaro es solo un ejemplo. El mismo sistema se aplica a cualquiera de los otros idiomas en este léxico.

El propósito de este libro es ayudar al viajero herbal. Desde estudiantes hasta biólogos profesionales en el campo, minoristas herbarios y mayoristas, personas que viven fuera de su propio país y herbolarios médicos. Principalmente me he limitado a las hierbas que crecen en Europa y el Mediterráneo, pero he incluido algunas del resto del mundo que se usan comúnmente en Europa.

Para terminar, creo que este léxico herbal será muy útil, no solo para Europa y el Mediterráneo, sino también para Asia, Australia y América.

Come usare il Lessico

Se parlate Italiano e volete sapere la parola ungherese per Borsa del pastore, andate all'indice Italiano nella seconda sezione e cercate Borsa del pastore. Vicino troverete un numero, in questo caso il 137. Poi andate al numero 137 nella prima parte e sotto il nome Latino *Capsella Bursa* e accanto a la lettera **H** vedrete Pásztortáska che è il nome ungherese per Borsa del pastore. Se conoscete solo il nome botanico comminciate con la prima sezione dove le piante sono elencate in ordine alfabetico sotto i loro nomi in Latino e sotto il nome della pianta nelle varie lingue.

E – Inglese; **F** – Francese; **G** – Tedesco; **S** – Svedese; **Sp** – Espagnolo;
I – Italiano; **Gr** – Greco; **H** – Ungherese; **P** – Polonese; **T** – Turco.

L'ungherese è solo un esempio. Lo stesso sistema si applica a qualsiasi altra lingua in questo Lessico.

Lo scopo di questo libro è quello di aiutare l'erborista. Dagli studenti ai biologi professionali nel proprio campo, dai dettaglianti ai grossisti, persone che vivono lontano dal loro paese e medici erboristisi. Sono riferito principalmente alle erbe che crescono in Europa e nel Mediterraneo ma ho incluso alcune dal resto del mondo che sono normalmente usate in Europa.

In conclusion, penso che questo Lessico Erbale sarà molto utile, non solo per l'Europa e il mediterraneo ma anche per l'Asia, Australia e le Americhe.

Πώς να χρησιμοποιήσετε το Λεξικό

Εάν είστε Έλληνας και θέλετε να μάθετε την ουγγρική λέξη για το *Καπσέλλα*, πηγαινεται στο Part Two, στον ελληνικό δείκτη, και βρείτε το *Καπσέλλα*. Εκει θα βρείτε έναν αριθμό, στην περίπτωση αυτή 137. Στη συνέχεια, πηγαίνετε στον αριθμό 137 στο Part One και κάτω από τη λατινική ονομασία *Capsella bursa*, στο γραμμα **H**, θα δείτε την *Pásztortáska* που είναι το ουγγρικό όνομα για το *Καπσέλλα*. Αν γνωρίζετε μόνο το βοτανικό όνομα πηγαίνετε στο Part One (Πρώτο Μέρος) όπου τα φυτά παρατίθενται αλφαβητικά με τα λατινικά τους ονόματα ακολουθουμενα απο το όνομα του φυτού στις διάφορες περιερχόμενες γλώσσες.

E – Αγγλικά; **F** – Γαλλικά; **G** – Γερμανικά; **S** – Σουηδικά; **Sp** – Ισπανικά; **I** – Ιταλικά; **Gr** – Ελληνικά; **H** – Ουγγρικά; **P** – Πολωνικά; **T** – Τουρκικά.

Τα ουγγρικά χρησιμοποιουνται ως παραδειγμα αλλα οι ιδιες διαδικασιες ισχυουν για οποιαδηποτε αλλη απο τις γλωσσες.

Ο σκοπός αυτού του βιβλίου είναι να βοηθήσει τον φυτικό ταξιδιώτη. Από φοιτητές έως επαγγελματίες βιολόγους στον τομέα, λιανοπωλητές βοτάνων και χονδρεμπόρους, άτομα που ζουν μακριά από τη χώρα τους και ιατρικούς βοτανολόγους. Καλύπτονται κυρίως βότανα που φυτρωνουν στην Ευρώπη και την Μεσόγειο, αλλά συμπεριλαμβάνονται και άλλα από τον υπόλοιπο κόσμο που χρησιμοποιούνται ευρέως στην Ευρώπη.

Κλείνοντας, πιστεύω ότι αυτό το Λεξικό θα ήταν πολύ χρήσιμο όχι μόνο για την Ευρώπη και τη Μεσόγειο αλλά και για την Ασία, την Αυστραλία και την Αμερική.

Hogyan használjuk a lexikont

Hogyha magyar anyanyelvű vagy és megszeretnéd tudni mi A *Pásztortáska* angol neve, akkor keresd meg a magyar indexet a második részben és találd meg "*Pásztortáska*". A szó mellett találsz egy számot, ebben az esetben 137.

Következő lépésként lapozz a 137-es számhoz az első részben. A latin név alatt (**Capsella Bursa**) az E betű mellet listázva megtalálhatod *Shepherd's Purse*, ami a *Pásztortáska* angol neve.

Amennyiben csak a Botanikai nevét ismered a növénynek, akkor menj az első részhez, ahol a növény neveket ábécérendben listázták a latin nevük szerint.

A latin név alatt megtalálod a növény többnyelvű listázását.

E – Angol. F – Francia. G – Német. S – Svéd. Sp – Spanyol. I – Olasz. Gr – Görög. H – Magyar. P – Lengyel. T – Török.

Ennek a könyvnek a célja, hogy segítse a hobbi botanikust. Tanulótól a biológus professzorig, gyógynövény árusoktól, nagykereskedőkig és akik messze élnek a saját hazájuktól.

Főként azok a gyógynövények találhatóak itt meg, amelyek Európában és a mediterrán térségben nőnek, de helyet kapott néhány az egész világból, amelyek Európában is használatosak.

Zárásképpen úgy érzem, hogy a Herbál lexikon nemcsak Európában és a mediterrán térségben, de Ázsiában, Ausztráliában és Amerikában is hasznos olvasmány lehet.

Jak korzystać z Leksykonu

J eśli jesteś polskim mówcą i chcesz poznać węgierskie słowo określające "Tasznik pospolity", zwróć się do polskiego indeksu w części drugiej i znajdź Tasznik pospolity. Obok znajdziesz numer, w tym przypadku 137. Następnie przejdź do numeru 137 w części pierwszej i poniżej łacińskiej nazwy *Capsella bursa*, a obok H zobaczysz Pásztortáską, która jest węgierską nazwą dla Tasznika. Jeśli znasz tylko nazwę botaniczną, przejdź do części pierwszej, gdzie rośliny są wymienione alfabetycznie pod ich łacińskimi nazwami, a poniżej znajduje się nazwa rośliny w różnych językach.

> **E** – angielski; **F** – francuski; **G** – Niemiecki; **S** – szwedzki; **Sp** – hiszpański; **I** – włoski; **Gr** – grecki; **H** – węgierski; **P** – polski; **T** – turecki.

Węgierski jest tylko przykładem. Ten sam system dotyczy dowolnego innego języka w tym Leksykonie.

Celem tej książki jest pomoc podróżnikom zielarskim. Od studentów do zawodowych biologów w terenie, zielarskich sprzedawców detalicznych i hurtowników, ludzi żyjących z dala od własnego kraju i medycznych zielarzy. Głównie skupiłam się na ziołach, które rosną w Europie i w basenie Morza Śródziemnego, ale także na tych z innych części świata, powszechnie używanych w Europie.

Mam nadzieję, że ten "Ziołowy Lexikon" będzie przydatny czytelnikom nie tylko z Europy i basenu Morza Śródziemnego, ale także z Azji, Australii i obu Ameryk.

Lexicon'u nasıl kullanıyoruz

Eğer anadili Türkçe olan biriyseniz ve 'Çoban çantası' kelimesinin Macarcasını merak ediyorsanız, İkinci Kısım (Part Two)'da bulunan Türkçe kelimeler fihristine gidip Çoban çantası kelimesini bulun. Kelimenin hemen yanında bir numara olacak, bu örnek için o numara 137. Sonra, Birinci Kısım (Part One)'da bulunan 137 numaraya gidin ve orada 'Capsella bursa' adlı Latince kelimenin altındaki listeden 'H' harfini seçince karşınıza Macarca 'Çoban çantası' anlamına gelen 'Pásztortáska' kelimesi çıkacak. Eğer sadece botanik ismi biliyorsanız tüm bitkilerin alfabetik sıralı olduğu Birinci Kısım'a gidin ve orada Latince kelimenin hemen altında bitkinin değişik dillerdeki karşılığını göreceksiniz.

E – İngilizce, F – Fransızca, G – Almanca, S – İsveççe, Sp – İspanyolca, I – İtalyanca, Gr – Yunanca, H – Macarca, P – Lehçe, T – Türkçe için.

Macarca sadece bir örnek. Ayni yöntem Lexicon'daki diğer tüm diller için de geçerli.

Bu kitabın amacı botanik seyyahlarına yardımcı olabilmektir. Alandaki öğrencilerden profesyonel biyologlara, toptan ya da perakende satış yapanlara, ülkelerinden uzakta bulunanlardan tıbbî bitki uzmanlarına kadar herkese. Çoğunlukla Avrupa'da ve Akdeniz'de yetişen bitkilere, fakat aynı zamanda dünyanın geri kalan kısmından olup Avrupa'da kullanılan bazı bitkilere de yer verildi.

Noktalarken, Herbal Lexixon'un yalnızca Akdeniz ve Avrupa için değil fakat Asya, Avusturalya ve Amerika için de faydalı olacağına inanıyorum.

PART I

THE HERBAL LEXICON

1. Abies alba
E. Silver Fir.
F. Sapin blanc
G. Weisstanne; Edeltanne
S. Silvergran
Sp. Abeto blanco
It. Abete bianco
Gr. Élato
Gr. Έλατο
H. Ezüst fenyő
P. Jodła pospolita
T. Dılber çam ağ.

2. Abies balsamea
E. Balsam Fir; Balm of
   Gilead Fir
F. Sapin baumier
G. Balsam-Tanne
S. Balsamgran
Sp. Abeto balsámico
It. Abete balsamico
H. Balzsam fenyő; Kanadai
   fenyő
P. Jodła balsamiczna
T. Balsam göknarı

3. Acacia catechu
E. Catechu Acacia; Black
   Catechu
F. Acacie cachou
G. Catechu Akazie
S. Katecuakacia
Sp. Acacia catechu
It. Catecù; Terracattù
Gr. Katetsoú
Gr. Κατετσού
H. Katechu-akácia
P. Akacja katechu
T. Kad hindi

4. Acacia nilotica
E. Gum Arabic; Acacia gum
F. Acacie du Sénégal; Acacie
   arabique
G. Gummi arabischer
S. Gummi arabicum
Sp. Goma arabica
It. Gomma arabica
Gr. Akakía i Senegálios;
   Aravikón kómmi
Gr. Ακακία η Σενεγάλιος·
   Αραβικόν κόμμι
H. Arab mézga; Gumiarabikum
P. Gumarabska
T. Beyaz zamk ağ.

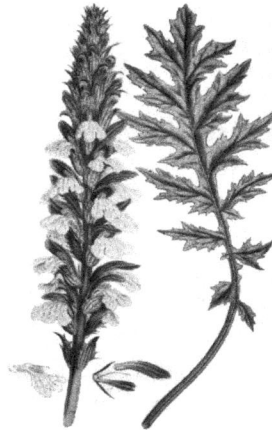

5. Acanthus mollis
E. Bearsbreech
F. Acanthe
G. Wahrer Bärenklau
S. Mjukakantus
Sp. Acanto
It. Acanto
Gr. Ákanthos; Apoúronos;
   Apriniá

Gr. Ἄκανθος· Ἀπούρονος·
  Ἀπρινιά
H. Medveltalp; Akantusz
P. Akant miękki
T. Ayı pençesı; Dikensiz
  kenger otu

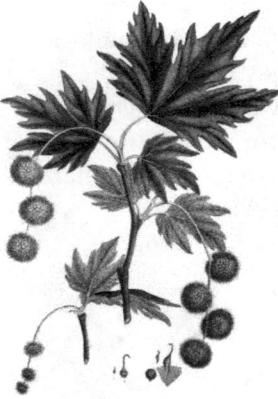

6. *Acer pseudoplatanus*
E. Sycamore
F. Sycomore
G. Berghorn
S. Tysklönn; Sykomorlönn
Sp. Sicomoro
It. Sicomoro
Gr. Sykomouriá; Psevdhoplátanos
Gr. Συκομουριά· Ψευδοπλάτανος
H. Hegyi juhar
P. Sykomor
T. Yalan ak ağ.

7. *Acer saccharum*
E. Sugar maple; Bird's eye maple
F. Érable à sucre
G. Zucker Ahorn
S. Silverlön
Sp. Arce; Maple
It. Acero

Gr. Sféndhamnos; Áker
Gr. Σφένδαμνος· Ἄκερ
H. Juhar
P. Klon srebrzysty
T. Kırmızı ısfenden ağ.

8. *Achillea millefolium*
E. Yarrow; Milfoil
F. Millefeuille; Achillée; Herbe à
  la coupure
G. Schafgarbe
S. Röllika
Sp. Milenrama; Milefolio
It. Achillea millefoglie
Gr. Achilléa; Chiliófilos
Gr. Αχιλλεία· Χιλιόφυλλος
H. Cickafarkkóró
P. Krwawnik pospolity
T. Cıvan perçsemi; Binbir yaprak

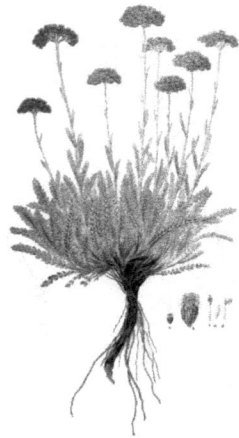

9. *Achillea ptarmica*
E. Sneezewort
F. Herbe à éternuer, Achillée
  sternutatoire
G. Sumpf-Schafgarbe;
  Bertam-Schafgarbe

S. Nysört
Sp. Camamila de muntanya
It. Ptarmica; Sternutella
Gr. Achillea i ptarnistikí
Gr. Αχιλλεία η πταρνιστική
H. Kenyérbél; Cickafark
P. Krwawnik kichawiec
T. Asırmak otu

10. *Aconitum napellus*
E. Aconite; Monkshood;
     Wolf'sbane
F. Aconit napel
G. Wolfswurz; Blauer Eisenhut
S. Stormhatt
Sp. Acónito; Tuera
It. Aconito
Gr. Akóniton; Striglóvotano
Gr. Ακόνιτον· Στριγγλοβότανο
H. Sisakvirág
P. Tojad mocny
T. Kaplan boğan

11. *Acorus calamus*
E. Sweet flag
F. Acore aromatique
G. Teichkalmus; Echter kalmus
S. Kalmus; Kalmusrot
Sp. Cálamo aromático; Acoro
It. Calamo aromatico
Gr. Ákoros
Gr. Ακορος
H. Kálmos
P. Tatarak zwyczajny
T. Eğır otu; Azak eğeri

12. *Actea spicata*
E. Black Baneberry
F. Actée en épis;
     Herbe de St Christophe

G. Christophskraut
S. Trolldruva
Sp. Cristobalina; Hierba de San
     Cristóbal
It. Barba di San Cristoforo; Actea
Gr. Aktéa
Gr. Ακτέα
H. Békabogyó
P. Czerniec gronkowy
T. Akta; Kristof otu

13. *Adiantum capillus-veneris*
E. Maidenhair fern; Venus hair
F. Adiante; Capillaire de
     Montpellier
G. Frauenhaarfarn; Venushaar
S. Venushär
Sp. Culantrillo; Capilaria
It. Capelvenere
Gr. Adhíanto; Polytríchi
Gr. Αδίαντο· Πολυτρίχι
H. Szent Ilona füve
P. Zanokcica kapilorek; Matki
     bożej włoski
T. Kinulcede; Baldırıkara

14. *Adonis aestivalis*
E. Summer Adonis
F. Adonide d'été; Goutte de sang
G. Adonis Sommerröschen;
     Feuerrröschen
S. Sommaradonis
Sp. Adonis de Verano; Gota de
     sangre
It. Adonide estive
Gr. Aghriopaparoúna; Adhonis o
     therinós
Gr. Αγριοπαπαρούνα· Άδωνις ο
     θερινός
H. Nyári hérics

P. Miłek letni
T. Yazlık kanavcı otu

15. *Adonis annua*
E. Pheasant's eye; Autumn
adonis
F. Adonide d'automne; Goutte de
sang
G. Herbstfeuerrröschen;
Blutsröpfchen
S. Höstadonis
Sp. Adonis de otuño
It. Adonide rossa
Gr. Moróhorto; Adhonis o
fthinoporinós
Gr. Μορόχορτο˙ Άδωνις ο
φθινοπωρινός
H. Hérics
P. Miłek jesien
T. Kanavcı otu

16. *Adonis flammea*
E. Flame Adonis
F. Adonis écarlate; Adonis
flamme
G. Brennendes Feuerröschen
Flammen-Adonisröschen
Sp. Ojo de faisán grande
It. Adonide scarlatta
Gr. Moróhorto
Gr. Μορόχορτο
H. Lángszinü-hérics
P. Miłek skarłatny
T. Cin lâlesi; Taç çiçeği

17. *Adonis vernalis*
E. False Hellebore; Spring
Adonis

F. Hellébore bâtard
G. Herbst-Adonisröschen
S. Våradonis
Sp. Eléboro falso; Adonis
Vernalis
It. Ellebore bastardo; Adonis
vernalis
Gr. Adhonis khimerinós;
Psevdhoellévoros
Gr. Άδωνις χειμερινός˙
Ψευδοελλέβορος
H. Tavaszi-hérics
P. Miłek wiosna
T. Avcı otu; Keklik gözü

18. *Aegopodium podagraria*
E. Ground Elder; Goutweed
F. Égopode podagraire; Herbe
aux goutteux
G. Geissfuss, gewöhnlicher
S. Kirskål
Sp. Hierba de San Gerardo
It. Girardina Silvestre; Podagraria
Gr. Egopódhio
Gr. Αιγοπόδιο
H. Kecsketalpfű
P. Podagrycznik
T. Keçi ayağı

19. *Aesculus hippocastanum*
E. Horse-chestnut
F. Marron d'Inde
G. Rosskastanien
S. Hästkastanj
Sp. Castaña de Indias
It. Castagno d'India; Ippocastano
Gr. Aghriokastaniá;
Ippokástanon

Gr. Αγριοκαστανιά·
Ιπποκάστανον
H. Vadgesztenye
P. Kasztan górzki,
Kasztanowiec
T. Yabani Kestane

19a. *Aetheorhiza palmata*→
Jateorhiza palmata

20. *Aethusa cynapium*
E. Fool's Parsley; Dog
Parsley
F. Faux persil; Petite ciguë
G. Hundspetersilie
S. Vild persilja
Sp. Apio de perro; Cicuta
menor
It. Prezzemolo velenosa
Gr. Ethúsa i kynápia
Gr. Εθούσα η κυνάπια
H. Mérges ádáz
P. Blekot; Szalej
T. Küçük subaldıran

21. *Agave americana*
E. Agave; Maguay; Century
plant
F. Agave d'Amérique
G. Agave Americana
S. Agave
Sp. Agave; Pita
It. Agave
Gr. Athánatos; Agávi
Gr. Αθάνατος· Αγαύη
H. Agavé
P. Agawa
T. Ağav

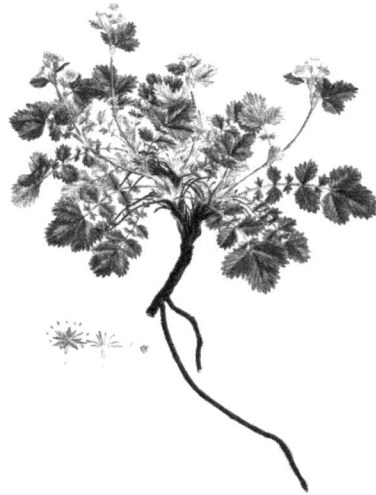

22. *Agrimonia eupatoria*
E. Agrimony
F. Agrimoine
G. Odermennig; Bruchwurz;
Lebenskraut
S. Småborre
Sp. Agrimonia
It. Agrimonia
Gr. Agrimónia; Asprozáki
Gr. Αγριμόνια· Ασπροζάκι
H. Közönséges párlófű; Apró
bojtorjan
P. Rzepik pospolity; Parzydło
T. Koyun otu; Kuzu pıtrağı; Adi
kızıl yaprak

23. *Agropyron repens*
E. Couchgrass
F. Chiendent
G. Quecke
S. Kvickrot
Sp. Grama

It. Gramigna; Caprinella
Gr. Agriádha
Gr. Αγριάδα
H. Tarackbúza
P. Perz
T. Ayrık otu; Nigil

23a. *Aetheorhiza palmata*→ *Jateorhiza palmata*

24. *Ajuga reptens*
E. Common Bugle
F. Bugle rampante
G. Günsel; Kreichender Günsel
S. Revsuga
Sp. Búgula
It. Bugula; Iva
Gr. Livanóhorta; Dhodhekánthio
Gr. Λιβανόχορτο˙ Δωδεκάνθιο
H. Indás infű
P. Dąbrówka
T. Dağ mayasıl otu

25. *Alchemilla alpina*
E. Alpine Lady's Mantle
F. Pied de lion; Alchémille des alpes
G. Alpen Frauenmantel
S. Fjällkåpa
Sp. Alquimila alpina; Pie de León
It. Alchemilla alpina
Gr. Leontopódhi
Gr. Λεοντοπόδι
H. Alpesi palástfű
P. Przywrotnik alpejski
T. Aslanpençesi otu (dağ)

26. *Alchemilla arvensis*
E. Parsley Piert; Breakstone; Colicwort

F. Perce-pierre; Alchémille des champs
G. Steinbrech; Gewöhnliche Ackerfrauenmantel
S. Jungfrukam
Sp. Alquimila arvense
It. Spacca pietra
Gr. Alchemilla i arouraía
Gr. Αλχεμίλλα η αρουραία
H. Ugari palástfű
P. Skrytek polny
T. Terspençe

27. *Alchemilla vulgaris*
E. Lady's Mantle
F. Manteau de Notre Dame; Alchémille
G. Frauenmantel
S. Daggkåpa
Sp. Alquimila
It. Alchemilla; Mantello della Madonna
Gr. Alchemílla i kiní
Gr. Αλχεμίλλα η κοινή
H. Palástfű
P. Przywrotnik
T. Aslan pençesı; Kirağiotu

28. *Aletris farinosa*
E. Unicorn root; Stargrass
F. Alétris farineux
G. Aletris,mehlige
S. Stjärngräs
Sp. Aletris
It. Aletris
Gr. Alétris
Gr. Αλέτρις
H. Aletris
P. Judrnia
T. Hartit

29. Alisma plantago

E. Water Plantain
F. Plantain d'eau; Flûteau
G. Froschlöffel
S. Svalting
Sp. Llanten de agua; Alisma
It. Piantaggine acquatica;
  Mestolaccia
Gr. Pendánevro tou neroú;
  Plemonóhorto
Gr. Πεντάνευρο τού νερού·
  Πλεμονόχορτο
H. Vízi hidor
P. Babka wodna
T. Çobandüdüğü

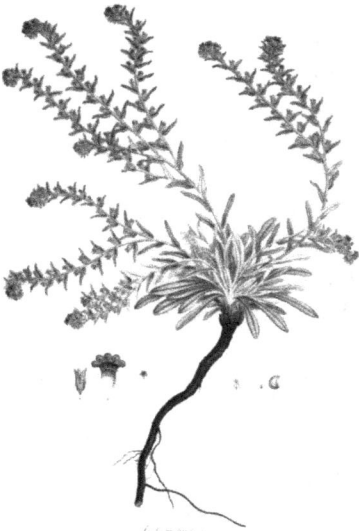

30. Alkanna tinctoria

E. Alkanet; Anchusa; Dyer's
  Bugloss
Fr. Orcanette; Alchanne; Buglosse
  officinale
G. Schminkwurz; Alkanna

S. Oxtunga
Sp. Alkana; Onoquiles
It. Alcanna
Gr. Vafórizo; Alkanníni
Gr. Βαφόριζο· Αλκαννίνη
H. Homoki pirosító
P. Alkanna
T. Havacı otu; Tüylü boya;
  Yerineği

31. Alliaria petiolata

E. Hedge Garlic; Mustard
  Garlic; Jack-by-the
  Hedge
F. Alliare officinale
G. Knoblauchsraukel;
  Lauchkraut
S. Löktrav
Sp. Aliaria; Hierba de ajo
It. Alliaria
Gr. Alliária; Stravánthi
Gr. Αλλιάρια· Στραβάνθι
H. Hagymaszagú zsombor;
P. Czosnaczek
T. Sarımsak hardalı; Sarımsak otu

32. Allium ascalonicum

E. Shallot
F. Échalote
G. Schalotte
S. Schalottenlök
Sp. Chalote; Cebollita
It. Cipollina
Gr. Esalót
Gr. Εσαλότ
H. Mogyoró hagyma; Salotta
  hagyma
P. Szalotka
T. Arpacik soğan

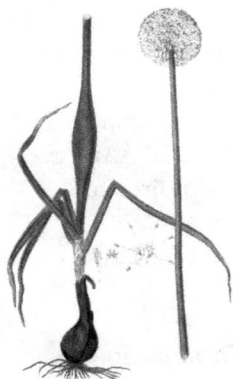

33. *Allium cepa*
E. Onion
F. Oignon
G. Zwiebel
S. Matlök
Sp. Cebolla
It. Cipolla
Gr. Kremídhi
Gr. Κρεμμύδι
H. Hagyma
P. Cebula
T. Soğan

34. *Allium porum*
E. Leek
F. Poireau
G. Lauch
S. Porjolök
Sp. Puerro
It. Porro
Gr. Prásso
Gr. Πράσσο
H. Póréhagyma
P. Por
T. Pırasa

35. *Allium sativum*
E. Garlic

F. Ail
G. Knoblauch
S. Vitlök
Sp. Ajo.
It. Aglio
Gr. Skórdho
Gr. Σκόρδο
H. Fokhagyma
P. Czosnek
T. Sarımsak

36. *Allium schoenoprasum*
E. Chive
F. Ciboulette; Civette
G. Schnittlauch
S. Gräslök
Sp. Cebollines; Ajo de puerto
It. Cipolla porraia; Erba cipollina
Gr. Skinóprason
Gr. Σκοινόπρασσον
H. Snidling; Metélőhagyma
P. Szczypiorek
T. Van bölgesinde kullanılır

37. *Allium ursinum*
E. Bear garlic; Ramsons
F. Ail des ours
G. Bärlauch; Wilder Knoblauch
S. Ramslök
Sp. Ajo de oso;
It. Aglio Ursino
Gr. Álio to arktikó
Gr. Ἅλιο τό αρκτικό
H. Medvehagyma
P. Czonek niedźwiedzi
T. Yabani sarımsak; Ayısarımsağı

38. *Alnus glutinosa*
E. Alder
F. Aulne

G. Schwarzerle
S. Klibbal
Sp. Aliso
It. Ontano
Gr. Sklíthra; Kléthra
Gr. Σκλήθρα˙ Κλέθρα
H. Éger
P. Olcha; Olsza
T. Kızıl ağ; Seyran ağ.

39. *Aloe vera*
E. Aloe vera
F. Aloé vera
G. Aloe
S. Såraloe; Äkta aloe
Sp. Áloe
It. Aloe
Gr. Alói; Alóchi
Gr. Αλόη˙ Αλόχη
H. Aloé
P. Aloes zwyczajny
T. Sarı Sabr; Öd ag.

40. *Aloysia triphylla*
E. Lemon Verbena
F. Verveine citronelle
G. Zitronenstrauch
S. Lippia
Sp. Hierba louisa
It. Verbena odorosa; Erba luisa;
    Cedrina
Gr. Louísa
Gr. Λουίζα
H. Citromkóró; Puncskóró
P. Cukrownica
T. Lipia

41. *Alpinia officinarum*
E. Galangal; Colic root
F. Galanga

G. Galanga
S. Galangarot
Sp. Galanga menor
It. Galanga
Gr. Galánga; Alpiniá
Gr. Γκαλάνγκα˙ Αλπινιά
H. Galanga gyökér
P. Galgant
T. Küçük havlıcan

42. *Althaea officinalis*
E. Marshmallow
F. Guimauve
G. Eibisch
S. Läkemalva
Sp. Malvavisco; Altea
It. Malva; Altea
Gr. Althéa; Neromolócha
Gr. Αλθέα˙ Νερομολόχα
H. Fehér mályva
P. Prawoślaz lekarski
T. Hatmi; Deli hatmi; İbiskökü

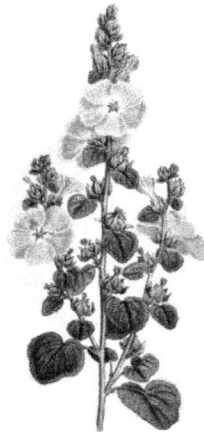

43. *Alcea rosea*
E. Hollyhock
F. Rose trémiere

G. Stockrose
S. Stockros
Sp. Malva Real; Barba de San
   Josep
It. Malvone; Altea fiori blu
Gr. Dhendromolókha
Gr. Δεντρομολόχα
H. Mályva rozsa
P. Prawoślaz ogrodny; Malwa
T. Gülhatmi çiçeği

44. *Amaranthum blitum*
E. Strawberry Blite; Wild
   Amaranth
F. Amarante blette
G. Gemeiner Erdamarant
S. Mållamarant
Sp. Bledos de comer
It. Blito; Amaranto selvatico
Gr. Vlíta
Gr. Βλήτα
H. Eperparéj
P. Szarłat rozpotarty
T. Hoşkıran otu

**45. *Amaranthus
hypochondriacus***
E. Love-Lies-Bleeding; Amaranth
F. Queue-de-renard; Amarante
G. Erdamarant; Fuchsschwanz
S. Toppamarant
Sp. Amaranto
It. Coda di Gatto; Amaranto
Gr. Amárantos
Gr. Αμάραντος
H. Csüngő amarant
P. Szarłat zwisły
T. Horoz ıbığı

46. *Amaranthus retroflexus*
E. Blite
F. Blette; Blède
G. Acker Fuchsschwanz
S. Svinamarant
Sp. Bledo
It. Blito; Amaranto spigato
Gr. Vlíta
Gr. Βλήτα
H. Eperparéj
P. Komosa
T. Yabani pazı

47. *Amni visnaga*
E. Khella; Amni-Visnaga
F. Amni-Visnage
G. Bischofskraut; Khella
S. Tandpetersilja
Sp. Biznaga; Escuradentis
It. Ammi Visnaga; Bisnaga
Gr. Khélla
Gr. Χέλλα
H. Fogpiszkálófü
P. Amni-Wisnaga
T. Diş otu; Hıltan; Kürdanotu

48. *Amygdala dulcis*
E. Almond
F. Amande
G. Mandel
S. Mandel
Sp. Almendra
It. Mandorla
Gr. Amýgdhalon
Gr. Αμύγδαλον
H. Mandula
P. Migdał
T. Badem ağ.

49. Anacardium occidentalis
E. Cashew Nut
F. Acajou
G. Kaschu Nuss; Nierenbaum
S. Elefantlus
Sp. Maranon; Anacardo
It. Acagiu
Gr. Akazoú
Gr. Ακαζού
H. Kesudió
P. Nanercz wschodni
T. Kaju; Amerika elması

50. Anagallis arvensis
E. Scarlet Pimpernel
F. Mouron rouge; Mouron des
    champs
G. Acker Gauchheil; Roter
    Gauchheil
S. Rödmire; Rödarv
Sp. Anagalide; Murajes
It. Anagallide
Gr. Anagális; Fellóhorta
Gr. Αναγκάλις· Φελλόχορτο
H. Mezei tikszem
P. Kurzyślep; Kursyśład polny
T. Sıçan kuluğı

51. Ananassa sativa
E. Pineapple
F. Anánas
G. Ananas
S. Ananas
Sp. Ananás;
It. Ananas
Gr. Ananás
Gr. Ανανάς
H. Ananász

P. Ananas
T. Ananas

51a. Anchusa officinalis→
Alkanna tinctoria

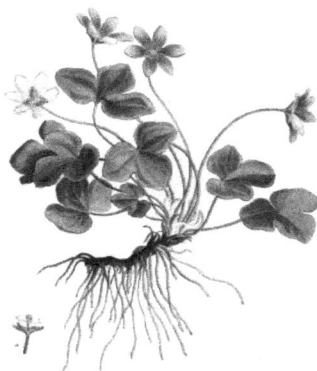

52. Anemone pulsatilla
E. Pasque flower; Pulsatilla
F. Pulsatille; Coquelourde; Fleur
    de pâques
G. Osterblume; Küchenschelle
S. Backsippa; Gökskälla
Sp. Pulsatila
It. Anemone pulsatilla
Gr. Poulsatílla
Gr. Πουλσατίλλα
H. Kökörcsin; Anemóna
P. Sasanka wiosenna; Sank
T. Rüzıgar çiç. Anemon

53. Anethum graveolens
E. Dill
F. Aneth
G. Dill; Gurkenkraut
S. Dill
Sp. Aneldo

It. Aneto
Gr. Anithos
Gr. Άνηθος
H. Kapor
P. Koper
T. Dere otu; Durak otu; Kötü
   kokulu rezene

54. Angelica archangelica
E. Angelica
F. Angélique
G. Angelika; Engelwurz
S. Kvanne
Sp. Angélica; Hierba del Santo
   Espiritu
It. Angelica Boemia
Gr. Agélika
Gr. Αγγέλικα
H. Angyalgyöker
P. Dzięgiel; Litwor
T. Melek otu

55. Aniba roseodora
E. Rosewood
F. Bois de rose
G. Rosenholz
S. Doftrosenträd
Sp. Palo de rosa
It. Legno di rosa
H. Amerikai rózsafa

56. Antennaria dioica
E. Catsfoot
F. Pied de chat; Antennaire
   dioïque
G. Katzenpfötchen
S. Kattfot
Sp. Pie de gatto; Cola de fuina
It. Zampa di gatto; Antennaria

Gr. Antennária
Gr. Αντεννάρια
H. Macskatalp
P. Ukwap dwupienny
T. Kedi ayağı

57. Anthemis nobilis
E. Roman Chamomile
F. Camomille romaine
G. Römische Kamille
S. Romersk kamomill
Sp. Manzanilla romana
It. Camomilla romana
Gr. Romaíkó hamomíli
Gr. Ρωμαϊκό χαμομήλι
H. Kamilla
P. Rumian szlachetny
T. Roman papatyası

58. Anthemis tinctoria
E. Dyer's Chamomile
F. Camomille des Teinturiers;
   Oeil-de-Boeuf
G. Faberkamille
S. Färgkulla
Sp. Ojo de buey
It. Camomilla per tintori
Gr. Anthémis i vafikí
Gr. Ανθέμις η βαφική
H. Festő pipitér
P. Rumian żółty
T. Boyacı papatyası

59. Anthoxanthum odoratum
E. Sweet Vernal Grass; Holy
   Grass
F. Flouve odorant;
   Gram d'olor

G. Mariengras; Gewöhnliches
   Ruchgras
S. Vårbrodd
Sp. Alestaz; Grama de Olor
It. Paleo odoroso
Gr. Anthóxantho
Gr. Ανθόξανθο
H. Borjúpázsit
P. Tomka wonna
T. Kokulu çayır otu

60. Anthriscus cerfolium
E. Chervil
F. Cerfeuil
G. Kerbel; Gewürzkerbel
S. Körvel
Sp. Cerefolio
It. Cerfoglio
Gr. Mironi; Skadzíki
Gr. Μυρώνι
    Σκαντζίκι
H. Turbolya
P. Trybułka, Trybula
T. Frenk maydonozu

61. Anthriscus silvestris
E. Cow Parsley
F. Persil d'âne; Cerfeuil
   sauvage
G. Waldkerbel
S. Hundkäx
Sp. Perejil de monte
It. Cerfoglio selvatico
Gr. Aghrio skadzíki
Gr. Άγριο σκαντζίκι
H. Erdei Turbolya
P. Trybułka lesna
T. Yabani frenk
   maydonozu

62. Anthyllis vulneraria
E. Kidney Vetch; Ladies
   Fingers
F. Anthyllide vulnéraire
G. Wundklee; Tannenklee
S. Getväppling
Sp. Vulneraria
It. Vulneraria
Gr. Anthýllis
Gr. Ανθύλλις
H. Réti nyúlhere
P. Prezłot pospolity;
   Welnica
T. Çoban gülü

**63. Aphanes arvensis→
Alchemilla arvensis**

64. Apium graveolens
E. Celery
F. Céleri
G. Seleri
S. Selleri
Sp. Apio
It. Sedano
Gr. Sélino
Gr. Σέλινο
H. Zeller
P. Selery
T. Kereviz

**65. Apocynum
androsaemifolium**
E. Bitter Root; Milkweed
F. Apocyn
G. Hundsgift
S. Flugkål
Sp. Apocinácea
It. Apocino

Gr. Apókinon to
   Andhrosemófilon
Gr. Απόκυνον το
   ανδροσαιμόφυλλον
H. Ebvész
P. Toina

66. Apocynum cannabinum
E. Dogbane; Canadian Hemp
F. Chanvre de Canada; Chanure
   indien
G. Hanfhundsgift
S. Indianhampa
Sp. Cañamo Indio; Apocino
It. Canapa Indiana del Canada
Gr. Apókynon to kanávion
Gr. Απόκυνον το κανάβιον
H. Ebdög
P. Toina konopna; Psia kapusta
T. Hint keneviri

67. Aquilegia vulgaris
E. Colombine
F. Colombine; Ancolie vulgaire
G. Waldakelei; Gemeine Akelei
S. Akleja
Sp. Aquileña; Clerigos bacabajo
It. Aquilegia
Gr. Aquiléghia
Gr. Ακουιλέγια
H. Harangláb; Sásfű
P. Orlik
T. Haseki küpesi

68. Arachis hypgaea
E. Peanut; Monkeynut;
   Groundnut
F. Cacahuète
G. Erdnuss
S. Jordnöt

Sp. Cacahuete; Mani
It. Arachide; Nocciolina
   americana
Gr. Arápiko fistíki
Gr. Αράπικο φυστίκι
H. Amerikai mogyoró
P. Orzacha podzeimna
T. Arap Fıstığı

69. Aralia racemosa
E. American Spikenard; Spignet
F. Anise sauvage; Aralie a
   grappes
G. Aralie
S. Lundaralia
Sp. Aralia
It. Aralia
Gr. Arália
Gr. Αράλια
H. Fürtös arália
P. Aralia

70. Arbutus unedo
E. Strawberry Tree
F. Arbousier
G. Erdbeerbaum
S. Smultronträd
Sp. Madroño; Albocero
It. Corbezzolo; Albatro
Gr. Koumariá
Gr. Κουμαριά
H. Szamócafá
P. Drzewo poziomkowe
T. Hoca yemeşi ağ; Adi
   kocayemiş

71. Arctium lappa
E. Burdock
F. Bardane
G. Klette

S. Stor kardborre
Sp. Bardana; Lampazo mayor
It. Bardana; Lappolone
Gr. Láppa; Kollitsídha
Gr. Λάππα· Κολλητσίδα
H. Bojtorján; Lapu
P. Łopuszno; Łopian większy
T. Büyük dulavret otu

72. *Arctostaphylos uva-ursi*
E. Bearberry
F. Raisin d'ours; Busserole
G. Bärentraube
S. Mjölon
Sp. Gayuba
It. Uva Ursina
Gr. Arkoudhostáphylo
Gr. Αρκουδοστάφυλο
H. Medveszőlő
P. Macznica lekarska
T. Ayı uzümü; Hoca yemişi

73. *Areca catechu*
E. Betelnut Palm
F. Aréquier; Cachou
G. Betelnusspalme; Arekanuss
S. Betelpalm
Sp. Areca; Bonga
It. Areca
Gr. Betél
Gr. Μπετέλ
H. Betel dió
P. Betel; Palma arekowa
T. Fufalağ; Arek hurma

74. *Arenaria rubra*
E. Sandwort; Sandspurry
F. Arénaire; Sabline
G. Sandkraut
S. Rödnarv

Sp. Arenaria roja
It. Arenaria; Spergola
Gr. Arenária
Gr. Αρενάρια
H. Pázsitlevelű homokhúr
P. Piaskowiec macierzankowy

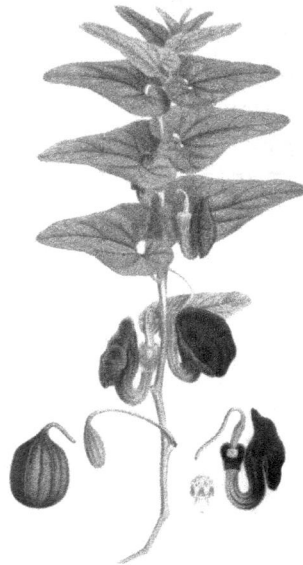

75. *Aristolochia longa*
E. Birthwort
F. Aristoloche clématite;
   Sarrasine
G. Osterluzei; Lange
   Hohlwurzel
S. Pipranka
Sp. Aristoloquia
It. Aristolochia; Strallogi;
   Erba stria
Gr. Aristolókhia;
   Bekroladhóchero
Gr. Αριστολόχια·
   Μπεκρολαδόχερο
H. Kígyogyökér

P. Smolnik; Korornak
powajnikowy
T. Loğusaotu (uzuyaprakli)

76. Aristolochia serpentaria
E. Snake Root
F. Aristoloche
G. Pfeifenwinde
Sp. Hierba de vibora
It. Serpentaria
Gr. Aristolókhia
Gr. Αριστολόχια
H. Serpentária gyökér
P. Kokornak
T. Zeravend

77. Armeria maritima
E. Thrift; Seapink
F. Œillet marin
G. Strandgrasnelke
S. Strandtrift
Sp. Armeria maritima
It. Armeria marittima
Gr. Armería; Halavóhorto
Gr. Αρμερία· Χαλαβόχορτο
H. Tengerparti pázsitszegfü
P. Zawciąg

78. Armoracia rusticana→
Cochliaria armoracia

79. Arnica montana
E. Arnica
F. Arnica; Tabac des Vosges
G. Arnika; Bergwohlverleih
S. Slåttergubbe
Sp. Árnica
It. Arnica; Tabacco di montagna
Gr. Arnikí

Gr. Αρνική
H. Árnika
P. Arnika; Pomornik
T. Arnika; Dağ tütünü

80. Artemesia abrotanum
E. Southernwood
Fr. Aurone; Garde-robe
G. Eberraute
S. Åbrodd
Sp. Abrótano; Boja
It. Abrotano
Gr. Pikrothámnos; Meletíni
Gr. Πικροθάμνος· Μελετίνη
H. Abruta Istenfa
P. Bylica boże drzewko
T. Kaysum

81. Artemesia absintium
E. Wormwood
F. Armoise; Absinthe
G. Wermut
S. Äkta malört
Sp. Ajenjo; Absintio; Arcacil
It. Assenzio Roano
Gr. Absithiá
Gr. Αψιθιά
H. Üröm
P. Bylica piołun
T. Pelin otu

82. Artemesia dracunculus
E. Tarragon
F. Estragon; Herbe du dragon
G. Estragon
S. Dragon
Sp. Estragón; Dragoncillo
It. Estragone; Dragoncello
Gr. Estragón; Strachoúri

Gr. Εστραγγόν˙ Στραχούρι
H. Tárkony
P. Dragonek; Estragon
T. Tarhun; Terğun

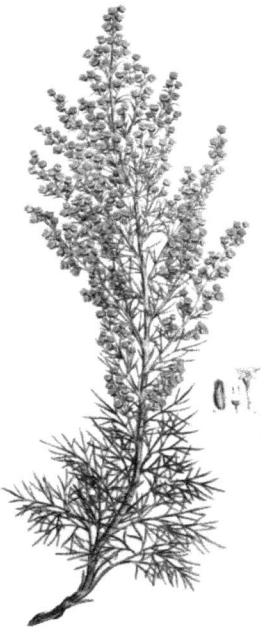

83. *Artemesia vulgaris*
E. Mugwort
F. Armoise commune
G. Mugwurz; Beifuss, gemeiner
S. Gråbo
Sp. Artemisa; Anastasia;
   Tomarajas
It. Artemisia volgare; Assenzio
   selvatico
Gr. Artemisía i kiní
Gr. Αρτεμισία η κοινή
H. Fekete üröm
P. Bylica pospolita
T. Ayvadana

84. *Arum maculatum*
E. Cuckoo pint; Lords and Ladies
F. Gouet maculé; Arum tacheté
G. Aronstab
S. Vanlig munkhätta
Sp. Aro
It. Gigaro macchiato
Gr. Áron; Fidhóhorto;
   Dhrakóntia
Gr. Άρον˙ Φιδόχορτο˙
   Δρακόντια
H. Foltos kontyvirág; Réti zsalya
P. Obraski plamiste
T. Yılan puçağı; Yılan yastıgı

85. *Arundo donax*
E. Giant Reed
Fr. Grand roseau
G. Pfahlrohr
S. Italieskt rör
Sp. Caña común; Carrizo
   junco
It. Canna comune
G. Kalámi
Gr. Καλάμι
H. Olasznád
P. Laskowa
T. Kargı kamışı

86. *Asarum europaeum*
E. Asarabacca; Wild Ginger
F. Asaret d'Europe; Herbe de
   Cabaret
G. Gewöhnliche Haselwurz
S. Hasselört
Sp. Ásaro; Oreja de fraile
It. Asaro; Baccaro
Gr. Asarón
Gr. Ασαρόν

H. Kapotnyak
P. Kropytnik
T. Avşar otu; Azaron

87. Asclepias tuberosa
E. Pleurisy Root
F. Asclépiade tubéreuse
G. Knollige Seidenpflanze
S. Orange sidenört
Sp. Algodon bulboso
It. Asclepiade
Gr. Asklipiós
Gr. Ασκληπιός
H. Gumós selyemkóró
P. Trojeść

88. Asparagus officinalis
E. Asparagus
F. Asperge
G. Spargel
S. Sparris
Sp. Esparago; Esparraguera
It. Asparago
Gr. Sparági
Gr. Σπαράγγι
H. Spárga
P. Szparag
T. Kuş konmaz

89. Asperula odorata
E. Sweet Woodruff
F. Aspérule odorante
G. Waldmeier; Meierkraut
S. Myskmadra
Sp. Asperula olorosa
It. Asperula odorosa; Raspello
Gr. Asperoúla
Gr. Ασπερούλα
H. Szagos Müge

P. Marzanka wonna
T. Kokulu yapişkan otu

90. Asphidosperma quebracho
E. Quebracho
F. Aspidosperme
G. Quebracho
S. Vit quebracho
Sp. Quebracho
It. Quebracho
H. Fehér kvebracsófa
P. Kebraczo białe.

91. Asphodelus ramosus
E. Asphodel
F. Asphodele
G. Asfodil
S. Afo diller
Sp. Albó
It. Asfodelo, Porraccio bianco
Gr. Asfódhelos
Gr. Ασφόδελος
H. Aszfodél
P. Asfodela; Złotogłów; Leliwa
T. Cırıs otu

92. Asplenium ceterach→ Ceterach officinarum

93. Astragalus canadensis
E. Astragalus; Milk Vetch
F. Astragal
G. Kanadischer Tragant
S. Kolvvedel
Sp. Astragalo
It. Astragalo vero
Gr. Astrágalos
Gr. Αστράγαλος
H. Csüdfű; Bokafű

P. Astragalus; Traganek
T. Çöven Kanada

94. Astragalus gummifer
E. Gum Tragacanth
F. Gomme Adragante
G. Tragant, Gummitragant
S. Dragantvedel
Sp. Astrágalo; Tragacento
It. Gomma adragante
Gr. Tragákantha
Gr. Τραγκάκανθα
H. Tragantmézga; Baktövis
P. Guma tragakanta
T. Kitre zamkı ag

95. Atriplex hortensis
E. Garden Orache
F. Arroche des jardins; Bonne
    dame
G. Melde; Wilder Spinat
S. Trädgårdsmålla
Sp. Armuelle; Almol
It. Atriplice; Spinacio selvatico
H. Kertilaboda; Labodaparéj
P. Łoboda ogrodowa
T. Talet; Tüld

96. Atropa belladonna
E. Belldonna; Deadly
    Nightshade; Dwale
F. Belladone
G. Tollkirsche; Wolfskirsche
S. Belladonna; Dvalbar
Sp. Belladonna; Solano.
It. Belladonna
Gr. Belladónna
Gr. Μπελλαντόννα
H. Nadragulya

P. Pokrzyk wilcza jagoda
T. Güzel avrat otu

97. Avena sativa
E. Oat
F. Avoine
G. Hafer
S. Havre
Sp. Avena; Sebada
It. Avena; Biada
Gr. Vrómi
Gr. Βρώμη
H. Zab
P. Owies
T. Yulaf; Ulaf

98. Azadirachta indica
E. Neem
F. Neem; Margosier
G. Niembaum; Neem
S. Neem
Sp. Nim; Neem; Nimbo de la
    india
It. Azadarac; Lillà d'India
Gr. Azádiracht
Gr. Αζάντιραχτ
H. Indiai lila; Nim
P. Miodła indyjska; Neem
T. Azadiraht; Tesbih ağ.

99. Ballota nigra
E. Black Horehound
F. Ballotte fétide; Ballotte noire
G. Stinkdom
S. Bosyska
Sp. Marrubio negro; Balota
    negra
It. Marrubio fetido; Ballota;
    Cimiciotta

Gr. Vromóhorta; Sidherolápatho;
    Valóti
Gr. Βρωμόχορτο·
    Σιδερολάπαθο· Βαλότη
H. Fekete peszterce
P. Mierznica czarna
T. Yalancı ısırgan; Kara yer
    pırasası; Kara ferasçyun

G. Bukkostrauch
S. Buchuruta
Sp. Buchú
It. Bucco
Gr. Varíosmos i vetouloidhís
Gr. Βαρίοσμος η βετουλοϊδής
H. Buchu
P. Gruczlin

100. Baptisia tinctoria
E. Wild Indigo
F. Indigo faux; Baptisia
    sauvage
G. Baptisie; Färberhülse
S. Gul färgväppling
Sp. Chirivita
It. Pratolino
Gr. Vaptoúsa
Gr. Βαπτούσα
H. Borsófürt
P. Dzikie indygo; Bratwa
    baptyska

101. Barbarea vulgaris
E. Yellow Rocket; Wintercress
F. Roquette
G. Ölrauke; Senfrauke
S. Sommargyllen
Sp. Roqueta común
It. Rughetta
Gr. Rókka
Gr. Ρόκκα
H. Tárkel; Kerti mustár
P. Gorczycznik pospolity;
    Rokieta-siewna
T. Roka; Nıcar otu

102. Barosma betulina
E. Buchu
F. Buchu

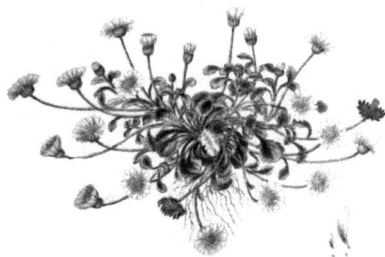

103. Bellis perennis
E. Daisy
F. Marguerite; Pâquerette
G. Gänseblümchen; Margerite
S. Tusenköna
Sp. Maya
It. Margheritina; Pratolina
Gr. Margharíta; Stekoúli
Gr. Μαργαρίτα· Στεκούλι
H. Margaréta; Százszorszép
P. Trwała; Stokrotka
T. Papatya çiç.

104. Berberis vulgaris
E. Barberry
F. Berbéris; Épine-vinette
G. Berberize
S. Berberis
Sp. Agracejo; Berberis
It. Berbero; Spina santa
Gr. Loutsiá; Vérveris;
    Oxyákanthos

Gr. Λουτσιά· Βέρβερις·
    Οξυάκανθος
H. Borbolya
P. Berberys
T. Diken üzümü; Amberbaris

105. Beta vulgaris
E. Beetroot
F. Bettereve
G. Runkelrübe
S. Beta
Sp. Remolacha
It. Barbabietola
Gr. Panzári
Gr. Παντζάρι
H. Répacukor
P. Burak
T. Çükündür; Pancar

106. Betonica officinalis
E. Wood Betony
F. Bétoine
G. Heil-Ziest; Echte Betonie
S. Humlesuga; Läkebetonica
Sp. Betonica
It. Betonica; Stregona
Gr. Betónika
Gr. Μπετόνικα
H. Orvosi tisztesfű
P. Bukwica lekarska
T. Tokalı çay; Kestere

107. Betula pendula
E. Siver Birch
F. Bouleau blanc
G. Birke
S. Vårtbjörk
Sp. Abedul; Albar
It. Betulla; Barancio
Gr. Simídha

Gr. Σημύδα
H. Nyir
P. Brzoza brodawkowata
T. Kokulu huş ağacı

108. Bidens tripartita
E. Burr Marigold; Water
    Agrimony
F. Bident; Cornuet
G. Zweizahn
S. Brunskära
Sp. Cañamo aquático; Paunga
It. Eupatorio acquatico
Gr. Neroagrimónia; Katafídhiá
Gr. Νεροαγριμόνια· Καταφιδιά
H. Subás farkasfog
P. Uczep; Dwuząb
T. Su keneviri

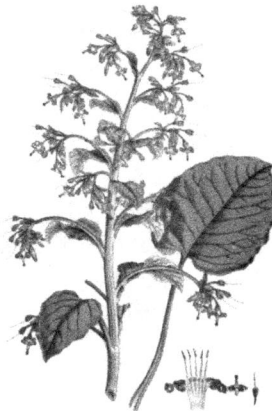

109. Borago officinalis
E. Borage
F. Bourrache
G. Borretsch
S. Gurkört
Sp. Borraja
It. Borragina; Borrana

Gr. Borádsa; Vóraghon
Gr. Μποράντσα˙ Βόραγον
H. Borrágófű
P. Ogórecznik
T. Zembil çiç.

110. Boswellia thurifera
E. Frankincense; Olibanum
F. Encens; Oliban
G. Weihrauch
S. Frankincenseträd;
  Olibanumträd
Sp. Incienso
It. Incenso
Gr. Liváni
Gr. Λιβάνι
H. Tömjén
P. Kadziło
T. Asılbend; Luban

111. Brassica alba
E. White Mustard
F. Moutarde blanche
G. Weisser Senf
S. Vitsenap
Sp. Mostaza blanca
It. Senape bianca
Gr. Lefkó sinápi
Gr. Λευκό σινάπι
H. Fehér mustár; Angol mustár
P. Gorczyca biala
T. Beyaz Hardal

112. Brassica botritis
E. Cauliflower
F. Chou-fleur
G. Blumenkohl
S. Blomkål
Sp. Coliflor

It. Cavolofiore
Gr. Kounoupídhi
Gr. Κουνουπίδι
H. Karfiol; Kelvirág
P. Kalafior
T. Karnabit; Karnıbahar

113. Brassica napus/oleifera
E. Rape; Coleseed
F. Colza
G. Winterraps; Öhlraps
S. Raps
Sp. Colza
It. Colza; Rapa coltivata
Gr. Eleokrámvi
Gr. Ελαιοκράμβη
H. Repce
P. Rzepak
T. Kolza

114. Brassica nigra
E. Black Mustard
F. Moutarde noire
G. Schwarzer Senf
S. Svartsenap
Sp. Mostaza negra
It. Senape nero
Gr. Mavro sinápi
Gr. Μαύρο σινάπι
H. Fekete Mustár
P. Gorczyca czarna
T. Kara Hardal

115. Brassica oleracea
E. Cabbage
F. Chou
G. Kohl
S. Kål
Sp. Col; Berza

It. Cavolo
Gr. Láchano
Gr. Λάχανο
H. Káposzta
P. Kapusta
T. Lahana

116. *Brassica rapa*
E. Turnip
F. Navet; Rave
G. Rübsen
S. Åkerkål
Sp. Nabo forajero
It. Rapa
Gr. Rápa; Ghogíli
Gr. Ράπα· Γογγύλι
H. Tarlórépa; Répa
P. Rzepik; Kapusta polna
T. Şalgam

117. *Brassica sinapistrum*
E. Mustard Greens; Charlock
F. Moutarde des champs; Sénevé
G. Wilder Senf; Acker-Senf
S. Åkersenap
Sp. Mostaza silvestre
It. Senape dei campi; Rapaccini
Gr. Ághrio sinápi; Vroúves
Gr. Βρούβες· Άγριο σινάπι
H. Vadrepce; Mustárrepcény;
  Mezei mustár
P. Świrzepa; Świerzop; Gorczyca
  polna
T. Yabani Hardal

118. *Brosimum alicastrum*
E. Breadnut Tree
F. Noyer à pain
G. Brotnussbaum

S. Brödnötsträd
Sp. Ramon
Gr. Vrisímo to alíkastro
Gr. Βρυσίμο το αλίκαστρο
H. Kenyérdiófa
P. Darzymlecznia

119. *Bryonia alba*
E. White Bryony
F. Bryone blanche
G. Schwarzbeerige Zaunrübe
S. Hundrova
Sp. Tuca; Nueza; Brionia
It. Brionia Bianca; Barbone
Gr. Vrionía i lefkí
Gr. Βρυωνία η λευκή·
  Αμπελουρίδα
H. Fekete földitök
P. Przestęp biały
T. Ak haylin

120. *Bryonia dioica/cretica*
E. Red Bryony
F. Bryone dioïque; Feu ardant;
  Vigne du diable
G. Rotbeerige Zaunrübe
S. Rod huntrova
Sp. Brionia; Alfesera; Carbasina
It. Fescera. Zucca selvatica;
  Brionia
Gr. Pondikostáfili
Gr. Ποντικοστάφυλο
H. Piros földitök
P. Przestęp dwupienny
T. Şeytan şalgamı

121. *Bupleurum falcatum*
E. Thorow-wax; Hare's Ear
F. Buplévre en faux

G. Sichel-Hasenohr
S. Harört
Sp. Mostacilla; Jaramango
It. Orecchio di lepre
Gr. Vouplévro
Gr. Βουπλέυρο
H. Kereklevelű bukákfű
P. Przewiercień okrą-gołistny
T. Tavşan kulağı; Çataltavşan

122. Buxus sempervirens
E. Box
F. Buis
G. Buchsbaum
S. Boxbum
Sp. Boj; Buje
It. Bosso
Gr. Pixári; Píxos
Gr. Πυξάρι· Πύξος
H. Buxus; Puszpáng
P. Bukszpan
T. Şimşir ağ.

123. Calamintha officinalis
E. Calamint
F. Calament
G. Bergminze
S. Stenkyndel
Sp. Calamento
It. Mentuccia; Nepitella
Gr. Kalamenta; Aghrioríghani
Gr. Καλαμέντα· Αγριορίγανη
H. Méhfű
P. Kalaminta; Czyścica
T. Misk otu; Yabani oğul otu

124. Calamus rotang
E. Rattan Palm
F. Rotang

G. Rattanpalme
Sp. Calamo
It. Canna d'India
Gr. Ratán; Indhikós kálamos
Gr. Ρατάν; Ινδικός κάλαμος
H. Rotáng pálma
P. Rotang palma
T. Hint kamışı

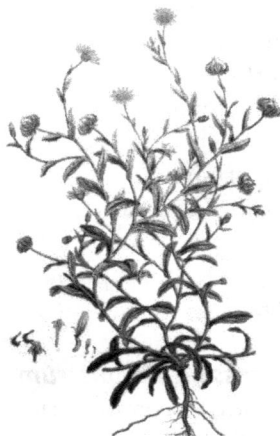

125. Calendula officinalis
E. Marigold; Pot Marigold;
F. Souci
G. Dotterblume; Ringelblume
S. Ringblomma
Sp. Maravilla; Caléndula; Rosa
   de muertos
It. Calendula; Fiorrancio
Gr. Kaléndoula;
   Nekrolouloúdho
Gr. Καλέντουλα·
   Νεκρολούλουδο
H. Körömvirág;
   Bársonyvirág
P. Nagietek lekarski
T. Aynısafa; Göze safa

126. Calla palustris
E. Water Arum; Bog Arum
F. Calle des marais
G. Drachenwurz;
   Schlagenkraut
S. Missne
Sp. Aro de agua
I. Calla palustre
Gr. Kálla i eloharís; Kalla i papía
Gr. Κάλλα η ελοχαρής˙ Κάλλα
   η παπία
H. Sárkánygyökér
P. Czermień
T. Yılanyastığıgiller;
   Kallazambağı

127. Calluna vulgaris
E. Heather; Ling
F. Bruyère; Callune
G. Heidenkraut; Erika
S. Ljung
Sp. Brecina; Brezo
It. Erica; Brugo
Gr. Érika; Kalloúna; Ághrio reíki
Gr. Έρικα˙ Καλλούνα ˙Αγριο
   ρείκι
H. Hanga; Erika; Csarab
P. Wrzos
T. Süpürge otu; Funda

128. Caltha palustris
E. Marsh Marigold
F. Populage; Souci des marais
G. Sumpfdotterblume
S. Kalvleka
Sp. Hierba centella
It. Calta palustre
Gr. Káltha i eloharís
Gr. Κάλθα η ελοχαρής
H. Mocsári gólyahír

P. Kaczeniec; Knieć błotna
T. Su nergisi; Lilpar

129. Calycanthus floridus
E. Carolina Allspice
F. Calycanthe; Arbre aux
   anémones
G. Gewürzstrauch
S. Hårig kryddbuske
Sp. Calicanto
It. Calicanto
Gr. Kalíkanthus i polyanthís
Gr. Καλίκανθος η
   πολυανθής
H. Fűszercserje
P.Woniał
T. Kadeh çiç; Kızıl çanak

129a. Calystegia sepium→
Convulvulus sepium

130. Camellia thea/Sinensis
E. Tea
F. Thé
G. Tee
S. Te
Sp. Té
It. Te
Gr. Tsái
Gr. Τσάϊ
H. Tea
P. Herbata
T. Çay

131. Campanula rapunculus
E. Rampion
F. Campanule raiponce
G. Rapunzel-Glockenblume
S. Rapunkelklocka
Sp. Rapinchos; Rapónchigo

It. Campanula; Rapunzolo
Gr. Kampanúla; Kodhónion i
  rápis
Gr. Καμπανούλα· Κωδώνιον η
  ράπις
H. Raponca
P. Dzwonek jednostronny
T. Büyük köklü çan çiçeği

132. Cananga odorata
E. Ylang-Ylang
F. Ylang-Ylang
G. Ylang-Ylang
S. Ilang-ilang
Sp. Ylang-Ylang
It. Ilang-Ilang
Gr. Yláng-Yláng
Gr. Υλάνγκ-Υλάνγκ
H. Ilang-Ilangfa
P. Ylang-Ylang
T. Yılang-Yılang; Kananga

133. Canarium commune
E. Elerni; Java Almond
F. Canarion; Elerni de Java
G. Elerni
S. Elemiträd
Sp. Canari; Almendra de Java
It. Elemi
Gr. Kanárion to kinó
Gr. Κανάριον το κοινό
H. Kanáridió
P. Kanarecznik
T. Kanariyon ağ.

134. Canella winterana
E. Wild Cinnamon
F. Canelle poivre
G. Weisse Zimt
S. Vit kanel

Sp. Canela silvestre
It. Canella selvatica
Gr. Ághria kanélla
Gr. Άγρια κανέλλα
H. Vad fahej; Fehér fahej
P. Cinamon biały
T. Yabani tarçın ağ

135. Cannabis sativa
E. Hemp
F. Chanvre
G. Hanf
S. Hampa
Sp. Cañamo común
It. Canapa
Gr. Kánnavis
Gr. Κάνναβις
H. Kender
P. Konopie swiene
T. Kınnab; Hint kınnabi; Kendir

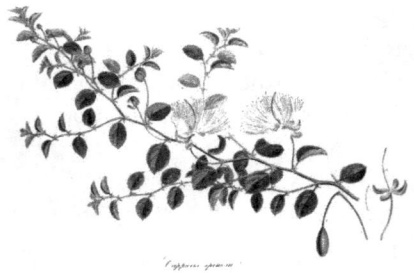

136. Capparis spinosa
E. Caper
F. Câprier
G. Kapern
S. Kapris
Sp. Alcaparra
It. Cappero
Gr. Káppari
Gr. Κάππαρη
H. Kapri

P. Kapar
T. Kebere; Keber fidanı

137. Capsella bursa-pastoris
E. Shepherd's Purse
F. Bourse-à-pasteur; Capselle
G. Hirtentäschel
S. Lomme
Sp. Bolsa de Pastor; Calzoncitos
It. Borsa di pastore; Bursa
    pastoris
Gr. Kapsélla; Kapsákio
Gr. Καπσέλλα˙ Καπσάκιο
H. Pásztortáska
P. Tasznik pospolity
T. Çoban çantası

138. Capsicum annuum
E. Sweet Pepper; Paprika; Green
    Pepper
F. Piment; Paprika
G. Spanischer Pfeffer; Paprika
S. Spansk peppar; Paprika
Sp. Pimiento
It. Peperone
Gr. Piperiá
Gr. Πιπεριά
H. Édés paprika; Piros paprika;
    Zöld paprika
P. Papryka
T. Kırmızı biber; Hint biberi

139. Capsicum frutescens/ Minimum
E. Cayenne Pepper; Chillie
    Pepper
F. Piment de Cayenne
G. Cayenne Pfeffer
S. Cayenne peppar
Sp. Pimiento de Cayenne

It. Pepe Cajenna; Capisco
Gr. Kayenne piperiá; Kaftí
    piperiá
Gr. Καγιέν πιπεριά˙ Καφτή
    πιπεριά
H. Erős paprika
P. Pieprz Kayenne
T. Acı biber

140. Cardamine amara
E. Bitter Cress
F. Cardamine amère
G. Bitteres Schaumkraut
S. Bäckbräsma
Sp. Berro amargo
It. Cardamine amara
Gr. Pikró kárdhamo
Gr. Πικρό κάρδαμο
H. Keserű kakukktorma
P. Rzeżucha gorska
T. Acıtere otu

141. Cardamine pratensis
E. Lady's Smock; Cuckoo Flower
F. Cardamine des prés; Cresson
    des prés
G. Wiesen-Schaumkraut;
    Kukucksblume
S. Ängsbräsma
Sp. Berro de prado
It. Cardamine; Billeri
Gr. Kardhamíni
Gr. Καρδαμίνη
H. Kakukktorma;
    Réti foszlár
P. Rzeżucha łąkowa
T. Çayır köpüktu

142. Carduus marianus→ Silybum marianum

143. Carex arenaria
E. Sandsedge
F. Laiche des sables; Carosse
G. Sand Segge; Riedgras
S. Sandstarr
Sp. Grama roja; Lastón
It. Carice
Gr. Arenária; Kíperi
Gr. Αρενάρια· Κύπερι
H. Tengerparti Sás
P. Turzyka; Dzieźega
T. Ayakotu

144. Carica papaya
E. Papaya; Papaw
F. Papaye; Arbre aux melons
G. Papaya
S. Papaija
Sp. Papayo
It. Papaia
Gr. Papaya
Gr. Παπάϊα
H. Papaya; Dinnyefa
P. Papaya; Melonowiec
T. Papaye

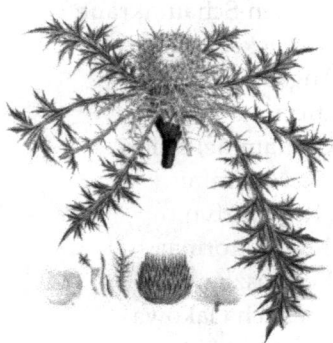

145. Carlina vulgaris
E. Carline Thistle
F. Chardon doré

G. Golddistel; Eberwurz
S. Spåtisel
Sp. Cardo carlino
It. Carlina comune
Gr. Karlína
Gr. Καρλίνα
Ar. Kharshûf barrî
Ar. خرشوف بري
H. Bábakalács
P. Dziewięćsił pospolity
T. Domuz dikeni

146. Carpinus betulus
E. Hornbeam
F. Charme
G. Hainbuche
S. Avenbok
Sp. Carpe común
It. Carpino
Gr. Kaprínos; Gavros
Gr. Καρπίνος; Γαύρος
H. Gyertyánfa
P. Grab
T. Gürgen ağ.

147. Carthamus tinctorius
E. Safflower
F. Carthame
G. Saflor; Fäberdistel
S. Safflor
Sp. Alazor; Cartamo;
    Azafranillo
It. Cartamo
Gr. Aghriozáfora; Saflanóni
Gr. Αγριοζάφορα·
    Σαφλανόνι
H. Pórsáfrány
P. Saflor; Krokosz barwierski
T. Aspir, Papağanyemi, Yalancı
    safran

148. Carum carvi
E. Caraway
F. Carvi; Cumin des prés
G. Kümmel
S. Kummin
Sp. Alcaravea; Carvi
It. Carvi; Cumino dei prati
Gr. Káron; Káro to kárvo
Gr. Κάρον· Κάρο το κάρβο
H. Kömény
P. Kminek; Karólek pospolity
T. Frenk kimyonu; Karaman
   kimyonu; Şifali kimyon

149. Cassia angustifolia
E. Senna
F. Séné
G. Sennesblätter;
   Sennestrauch
S. Senna
Sp. Sen
It. Cassia; Senna
Gr. Senna
Gr. Σεννά
H. Szennabokor
P. Senes
T. Sinameki; Sivri yapraklı
   sinameki

150. Cassia fistula
E. Indian Laburnum
F. Casse fistuleuse
G. Röhrenkassie
S. Rörkassia
It. Cassia canna macassar
Sp. Cañafistula
Gr. Kássia i indhikí
Gr. Κάσσια η ινδική
H. Mannakasszia
P. Senes cewkowaty

T. Hıyar-şenber ağ;
   Hint hıyarı

151. Castanea sativa
E. Sweet Chestnut
F. Châtaigne; Marron
G. Edelkastanie
S. Äkta kastanj
Sp. Castaño
It. Castagno
Gr. Kástano
Gr. Κάστανο
H. Gesztenye
P. Kasztan
T. Kestane ağ.

152. Catha edulis
E. Khat; Qat
F. Khat
G. Katstrauch; Bügelholz
S. Khat
Sp. Kaat; Té de Arabia
It. Cata
Gr. Kat
Gr. Κατ
H. Arabtea
P. Kata jadalna; Czuwaliczka
   jadalna
T. Kat; Arabistan çayı

**153. Caulophyllum
thalictroides**
E. Blue Cohosh; Squaw Root
F. Caulophylle
G. Frauenwurzel; Hahnenfuss
S. Azurbär
Sp. Cohosh azul
It. Caulofillo, Radice Indiana
H. Kék indiángyökér
P. Kaulofil

154. *Ceanothos americanus*
E. Red Root; New Jersey Tea
F. Ceonanthe d'Amerique
G. Säckelblume
Sp. Té de New Jersey
It. Ceanoto
Gr. Kéanthos o amerikanós
Gr. Κέανθος ο αμερικανός
H. Fehér táskavirág
P. Prusznik Amerykański;
   Herbata z New Jersey
T. Jersey çay ceonanthus

155. *Cedrus libani*
E. Cedar
F. Cèdre
G. Zeder
S. Cedar
Sp. Cedro
It. Cedro
Gr. Kédhros
Gr. Κέδρος
H. Cédrus
P. Cedrowy
T. Sedir; Lübnan çam ağ.;
   Lübnan sarvisi

156. *Ceiba pentandra*
E. Kapok; Silk Cotton Tree
F. Kapok; Arbre à coton
G. Kapok
S. Kapokträd, Glansull
Sp. Cieba de lana; Pochote
It. Sterculea
Gr. Kápok
Gr. Κάποκ
H. Kapokfa
P. Kapok
T. Kapok ağ

157. *Celtis australis*
E. Hackberry; Nettlewood
F. Micocolier de Provence
G. Südlicher Zurgelbaum
S. Europeisk bäralm
Sp. Almez; Lodonero
It. Bagolaro; Spaccasassi
Gr. Melikoukya; Keltis i notyas
Gr. Μελικουκιά; Κέλτις η νότιας
H. Déli ostorfa
P. Wiązowięc południowy
T. Adi çitlenbık; Yaygın çitlenbık

158. *Centaurea cyanus*
E. Cornflower; Bluebottle
F. Bluet
G. Kornblume
S. Blåklint
Sp. Azulejo; Aciano
It. Fiordaliso vero
Gr. Kentoúria; Bloué
Gr. Κεντούρια· Μπλουέ
H. Búzavirág
P. Bławatek
T. Mavi peyğamber çiç.

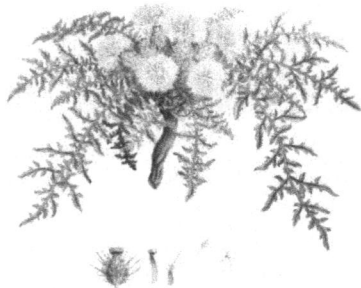

159. *Centaurea scabiosa*
E. Knapweed
F. Centaurée scabieuse

G. Skabiosen-Flockenblume
S. Väddklint
It. Fiordaliso vedovina; Erba di San Barnabo
Sp. Gratabous
Gr. Kentauria i skabióza
Gr. Κενταύρια η σκαμπιόξα
H. Vastövű imola
P. Chaber drakiewnik

160. Centaurium erythraea
E. Centuary; Feverwort
F. Petite centaurée
G. Tausendguldenkraut
S. Flockarun
Sp. Centaurea
It. Centaurea minore; Biondella
Gr. Thermóhorto; Kininóhorto
Gr. Θερμόχορτο· Κινινόχορτο
H. Ezerjófű; Százforintfű
P. Centauria zwyczajna
T. Kantaryon

161. Centella asiatica→
Hydrocotyle asiatica

162. Centranthus ruber
E. Red-Spur Valerian
F. Valériane rouge; Lilas d'Espagne
G. Spornblume
S. Flerårig pipört
Sp. Valeriana roja
It. Valeriana rossa
Gr. Análatos; Moscholiós
Gr. Ανάλατος; Μοσχολιός
H. Piros valerian
P. Ostrogowiec czerwony
T. Kırmızı kedi otu

163. Cephaelis ipecacuanha
E. Ipecacuanha
F. Ipécacuana
G. Ipekakuana; Brechwurzel
S. Kräkrot
Sp. Ipecacuana
It. Ipecacuana
Gr. Ipekakuána; Ipéka
Gr. Ιπεκακουάνα· Ιπέκα
H. Ipkakuána
P. Ipekakuana

164. Ceratonia siliqua
E. Carob Bean; Locust Bean
F. Caroube
G. Johannisbrot
S. Johannesbrödträd
Sp. Algarroba
It. Carrube
Gr. Haroúpi
Gr. Χαρούπι
H. Szentjánoskenyér
P. Chleb Świetojański
T. Keçi buynuzu ağ.

165. Ceterach officinarum
E. Common Spleenwort; Rusty-back Fern
F. Cétérach; Doradille
G. Schriftfarn
S. Mjältbräken
Sp. Doradilla
It. Spaccapietra; Erba dorata
Gr. Tséterach; Skorpídhi; Chrisóhorta
Gr. Τσέτερακ· Σκορπίδι· Χρυσόχορτο
H. Pikkelypáfrány

P. Śledzionka skalna
T. Altın otu

166. Cetraria islandica
E. Iceland Moss
F. Lichen d'Islande; Mousse d'Islande
G. Isländisches Moos; Brocken Moos
S. Islandslav
Sp. Liquen de Islandia
It. Lichene Islandico
Gr. Tsetrária
Gr. Τσετράρια
H. Izlandi zuzmó
P. Płutnica islanzka
T. İslanda likeni; İslanda yoğsunu

167. Chamaenarion angustifolium→ Epilobium angustifolium

168. Chamomilla suaveolens
E. Pineapple Weed
F. Herbe anánas
G. Strahllose Kamille
S. Gatkamomill
Sp. Magarza menor
It. Camomilla falsa; Erba ananas
H. Sugártalan székfű
P. Rumianek bezpromieniowy

169. Cheiranthus cheiri
E. Wallflower
F. Giroflée; Violier
G. Goldlack
S. Gyllenlack: Kårel
Sp. Alhelí
It. Violacciocca
Gr. Kítrini violétta; Manitiá

Gr. Κίτρινη βιολέττα· Μανιτιά
H. Sárga viola; Téli viola
P. Lak pospolity
T. Sarı şebboy

170. Chelidonium majus
E. Greater Celandine
F. Grande chélidoine
G. Schöllkraut
S. Skelört
Sp. Celidonia
It. Erba da porri; Chelidonia maggiore
Gr. Helidhónion
Gr. Χελιδόνιον
H. Vérehulló fecskefű; Vérfű
P. Glistnik; Jaskólcze ziele
T. Kırlangıc otu; Büyük halile

171. Chelone glabra
E. Balmoney
F. Chélonée; Galane
G. Schildblume
S. Vit sköldpaddsört
Sp. Cabeza de tortuga
It. Galana spicata
Gr. Chelóni i lía
Gr. Χελόνη η λεία
H. Kopasz gerlefey
P. Żółwik nagi
T. Tosbaği çiç.

172. Chenopodium album
E. Fat Hen; White Goosefoot
F. Patte d'oie blanc
G. Weisser Gänsefuss
S. Svinmålla
Sp. Cenizo; Berza perruna
It. Farinaccio; Farinello commune
Gr. Aghrio spánaki

Gr. Ἄγριο σπάνακι
H. Kövér tyúk
P. Komosa biała
T. Ak pazıs

173. Chenopodium ambrosiodes

E. Wormseed; Jerusalem Tea
F. Ambroisine; Thé du Mexique
G. Wurmsamen; Traubenkraut
S. Maskmålla
Sp. Pazote; Santonico; Epazote; Paico
It. Santonica; Semenzina ambrosia
Gr. Chinopódhion to ambrosioïdhes
Gr. Χηνοπόδιον το αμπροσιοειδές
H. Mirha libatop
P. Komosa piżmowa
T. Yayla çiç. Meksika çayı

174. Chenopodium bonus-henricus

E. Good King Henry; Goosefoot; All Good
F. Bon-Henri
G. Guter Heinrich
S. Lungrot
Sp. Zurrón; Pie de ganso; Anserina
It. Farinello buon-enrico
Gr. Aghrio spánaki
Gr. Ἄγριο σπάνακι
Ar. Kulluh tayab
Ar. كله طيب
H. Libatalp; Vadparéj; Kenófű
P. Komosa strzałkowata
T. Yabani asfanak; Yabani ıspanak

175. Chimaphila umbellata

E. Spotted Wintergreen; Pipissewa
F. Herbe d'hiver
G. Harnkraut
S. Ryl
Sp. Quimafila
It. Chimafila
Gr. Chimaefilo
Gr. Χειμαίφιλο
H. Ernyőskörtike
P. Pomocnik
T. Kekliküzümü

176. Chionanthus virginicus

E. Fringe Tree
F. Chionanthe; Arbre de neige
G. Schneeflockenstrauch
S. Snöflockbuske
Sp. Quiónanto
It. Chionanto
Gr. Kiónanto
Gr. Κιόναντο
H. Amerikai hópehelyfa
P. Śniegowiec wirginijski
T. Püskül ağacı

177. Chlorophlora tinctoria

E. Yellow Wood
F. Mûrier des teinturiers
G. Färbermaulbeerbaum
S. Fustikträd
Sp. Dinde
It. Legno giallo, Legno citrico
Gr. Chlorofora i vaftiki
Gr. Χλωροφλωρά η βαφτική
H. Sárga virgilia
P. Przekipień

178. Chondros crispus

E. Irish moss; Carragheen moss

F. Chondre crépu; Carragheen
G. Irisches Moos
S. Karragentång
Sp. Algas Irlandesas; Lichene
Carragaen
It. Carragenina; Lichene
Carrageen
Gr. Karághinon; Hóndhros o
polýmorphos
Gr. Καράγινον· Χόνδρος ό
πολύμορφος
H. Gyöngyös tengeri moszat
P. Chrząstnik
T. İrlanda yosunu

**178a. Chrysanthemum
cinerarifolium→ Tanacetum
cinerarifolium**

**179. Chrysanthemum
leucanthemum**
E. Ox-eye Daisy
F. Grande pâquerette
G. Magerwiesen-Margerite
S. Prästktage
Sp. Margarita común
It. Margherita dei prati
Gr.Tsitsimídha; Ághria
mandhilídha
Gr.Τσιτσιμίδα· Άγρια
μανδιλίδα
H. Réti margitvirág
P. Złocien właściwy
T. Çayır papatyası

**180. Chrysanthemum vulgare→
Tanacetum vulgare**

181. Cicer arietinum
E. Chickpea; Garbanzo Bean

F. Pois chiche
G. Kichererbse
S. Kikärt
Sp. Garbanzo
It. Cecci
Gr. Revíthi
Gr. Ρεβίθι
H. Csicseriborsó
P. Ciecierzyca
T. Nohud

182. Cichorium endivia
E. Endive
F. Endive; Scarole
G. Endivie
S. Endivia
Sp. Escarol
It. Indivia
Gr. Andíthi
Gr. Αντίδι
H. Endivia; Salátakatáng
P. Endywia
T. Kıvırcık hindiba

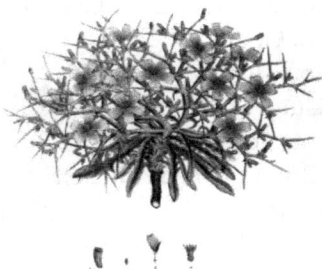

183. Cichorium intybus
E. Chicory; Succory
F. Chicorée
G. Zichorie; Wegwarte
S. Cikoria
Sp. Achicoria amarga
It. Cicoria

Gr. Pikralídha; Pikromároulo;
   Kíchori
Gr. Πικραλίδα˙ Πικρομάρουλο˙
   Κίχορι
H. Mezei Katáng
P. Cykoria
T. Citlik; Hindiba, Yaban
   marulu

184. Cicuta virosa
E. Cowbane
F. Ciguë aquatique
G. Wasserschierling
S. Sprängört
Sp. Cicuta acuatica;
   Cicuta virosa
It. Cicuta acquatica
Gr. Psevdhokónio;
   Kikoúta
Gr. Ψευδοκώνειο˙ Κικούτα
H. Gyilkos csomorika
P. Cykuta jadowita; Szalej
   jadowity
T. Su Baldıranı

185. Cimicifuga racemosa
E. Black Cohosh
F. Cimicaire; Cimicifuga
G. Schwarzes Schlangelwurzel;
   Trauben-Silberkerze
S. Silverax
Sp. Cimicifuga
It. Cimicifuga
Gr. Simitsifoúga
Gr. Σιμιτσιφούγκα
H. Poloskafű
P. Pchlica; Pluskwica
T. Karayılan otu

186. Cinchona calysaya
E. Cinchona; Calysaya
F. Quinquin jaune
G. Chinarindenbaum, gelber
S. Kinatrad
Sp. Quina calisaya
It. China calisaia
Gr. Kína
Gr. Κίνα.
H. Kínafa
P. Chinowiec
T. Knakna ağ.

187. Cinnamomum camphora
E. Camphor
F. Camphre
G. Kampfer
S. Kamferträd
Sp. Alcanfor
It. Canfora
Gr. Kámphora
Gr. Κάμφορα
H. Kámfor
P. Kamfora
T. Kâfuru

188. Cinnamomum cassia
E. Cassia
F. Casse
G. Chinesischer Zimt
S. Kassiakanel
Sp. Canela China
It. Canella China
Gr. Kássia
Gr. Κάσσια
H. Kasszia
P. Kasja
T. Saliha; Yalan tarçın ağ.

189. *Cinnamomum zeylanicum*
E. Cinnamon
F. Canelle
G. Zimt
S. Äkta kanel
Sp. Canelo
It. Canella
Gr. Kanélla
Gr. Κανέλλα
H. Fahéj
P. Cynamon
T. Tarçın ağ. Kurfa ağ

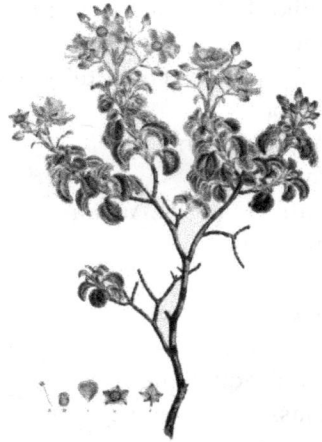

190. *Cirsium arvensis*
E. Creeping Thistle.
F. Chardon des champs; Cirse des champs
G. Ackerdistel
S. Åkertistel
Sp. Cardo cunidor; Cardo olorosa
It. Cardo campestre
Gr. Kírsion to arouraíon
Gr. Κίρσιον το αρουραίον
H. Mezei Bogáncs
P. Ostrożeń polny

191. *Cirsium vulgare*
E. Spear Thistle
F. Cirse Vulgaire
G. Gemeine Kratzdistel
S. Vägtistel
Sp. Cardo borriquero
It. Cardo asinine
Gr. Kírsion to kínon
Gr. Κίρσιον το κοινόν
H. Bogáncs
P. Ostrożeń lancetowaty

192. *Cistus incanus*
E. Pink Rockrose
F. Helianthéme
G. Zistrose
S. Grå cistros
Sp. Helintemo
It. Cisto incano
Gr. Kounoúkla; Kistós
Gr. Κουνούκλα· Κιστός
H. Bodor rózsa
P. Róża pszczelna
T. Tüylü laden

193. *Cistus ladinifer*
E. Gum Rockrose
F. Ciste ladanifère; Lédon
G. Gummizistrose
S. Ladanumcistros
Sp. Jara; Estepa
It. Ladano; Cisto l adinifero
Gr. Ládhano
Gr. Λάδανο
H. Gumi bodor rózsa

P. Czystk guma
T. Laden

194. Citrullus vulgaris
E. Watermelon
F. Pastèque; Melon d'eau
G. Wassermelone; Arbuse
S. Vattenmelon
Sp. Sandia
It. Anguria
Gr. Karpoúzi
Gr. Καρπούζι
H. Görögdinnye
P. Kawon; Arbuz
T. Karpuz

195. Citrus aurantifolia
E. Lime
F. Lime; Citron vert
G. Limette
S. Lime
Sp. Lima
It. Limetta
Gr. Lime; Moscholemoniá
Gr. Λαίμ˙ Μοσχολεμονιά
H. Trópusi citrom
P. Lima
T. Misket limonu

196. Citrus aurantium
E. Bitter Orange
F. Bigarade; Orange amère
G. Bitterorangen; Pommeranzen
S. Pomerans
Sp. Naranjo amargo
It. Arancio amaro; Cetrangolo
Gr. Neránzi
Gr. Νεράντζι

H. Keserű narancs
P. Pomarańcza gorzka
T. Turunc ağ.

197. Citrus bergamia
E. Bergamot Orange
F. Bergamote
G. Bergamotte
S. Bergamott
Sp. Bergamoto; Toronjo
It. Bergamotto
Gr. Perghamóto
Gr. Περγαμότο
H. Bergamott-narancs
P. Bergamoto
T. Bergamot ağ.

198. Citrus limonum
E. Lemon
F. Citron
G. Zitrone
S. Citron
Sp. Limon
It. Limone
Gr. Lemóni
Gr. Λεμόνι
H. Citrom
P. Cytryna
T. Limon

199. Citrus paradisi
E. Grapefruit
F. Pamplemousse
G. Pampelmuse
S. Grapfrukt
Sp. Pamplemusa
It. Pompelmo
Gr. Grapefrout

Gr. Γρέιπφρουτ
H. Citrancs; Grépfruit
P. Grejpfrut
T. Greyfurt

200. *Citrus reticulata*
E. Mandarin
F. Mandarine
G. Mandarine
S. Mandarin
Sp. Mandarina
It. Mandarina
Gr. Mandarini
Gr. Μανταρίνι
H. Mandarin
P. Mandarynka
T. Mandarına; Çin portokal

201. *Citrus sinensis*
E. Orange
F. Orange
G. Orange
S. Apelsin
Sp. Naranjo dulce
It. Arancio dolce
Gr. Portokáli
Gr. Πορτοκάλι
H. Narancs
P. Pomaráncza
T. Portokal; Portakal

202. *Claviceps purpurea*
E. Ergot
F. Ergot de seigle
G. Mutterkorn; Roggenmutter
S. Myöldryga
Sp. Cornezuelo; Espolon
It. Grano esperonata
Gr. Ergótion; Ghomfofóros

Gr. Εργότιον· Γομφοφόρος
H. Anyarozs
P. Sporysz; Buławinka czerwona
T. Çavdar mahmuzu

203. *Clemetis vitalba*
E. Traveller's Joy; Old Man's
Beard
F. Clématite des haies; Barbe du
vieillard
G. Waldrebe
S. Skogsklematis
Sp. Clemátide; Hierba de los
pordioseros
It. Clemátide flámula; Vitalba
clematis
Gr. Agrabelidha; Klimatsídha
Gr. Αγραμπελίδα· Κλιματσίδα
H. Közönséges iszalag
P. Powojnik pnacy
T. Peçek; Filbahar; Akasma (adi)

204. *Cnicus benedictus*
E. Blessed Thistle; Holy Thistle
F. Chardon bénit; Cnicaut
bénit
G. Bitterdistel; Benediktenkraut
S. Kardbenedikt
Sp. Cardo santo
It. Cardo santo; Cardo
benedetto
Gr. Kníkous; Kardhosánto;
Ayágatho
Gr. Κνίκους· Καρδοσάντο·
Αγιάγκαθο
H. Szentelt bogáncs
P. Karda Benedykta; Drapacz
lekarski
T. Mübarek dikenı; Şevket otu

205. Cochlearia amoracia
H. Horseradish
F. Raifort
G. Meerrettich
S. Pepparot
Sp. Rábano picante; Armoracia
It. Barbaforte; Rápano
Gr. Chréno
Gr. Χρένο
H. Torma
P. Chrzan
T. Bayır turpu; Siyah torpu

206. Cochlearia officinalis
E. Scurvy Grass
F. Cochléaria
G. Löffelkraut
S. Skörbjuggsört
Sp. Coclearia; Totes
It. Coclearia
Gr. Kochliáris i
    pharmakeftikí
Gr. Κοχλιάρις η φαρμακευτική
H. Kalánfű
P. Warzucha lekarska
T. Kaşık otu

207. Cocos nucifera
E. Coconut
F. Noix de coco
G. Kokospalme
S. Kokospalm
Sp. Coco
It. Noce di cocco
Gr. Indhikí karídha
Gr. Ινδική καρύδα
H. Kókuszdió
P. Kokos
T. Hindistan cevizi; Narcıl

208. Coffea arabica
E. Coffee
F. Café
G. Kafee
S. Kaffe
Sp. Café
It. Caffè
Gr. Kafés
Gr. Καφές
H. Kávé
P. Kawa
T. Kahve

209. Cola nitida
E. Kola Nut
F. Kola; Café du Sudan
G. Kolanuss
S. Kolaträd
Sp. Cola
It. Cola; Noce di Sudan
Gr. Kóla; Karíon tis kólas
Gr. Κόλα· Καρύον της κόλας
H. Kóla
P. Kola błyszcząca
T. Zinc cevizi; Kola cevizi

210. Colchicum autumnale
E. Autumn Crocus; Meadow
    Saffron
F. Colchique d'automne
G. Herbstzeitlose
Sp. Colchico; Cólquico
S. Tidlösa
It. Zafferano falso; Colchico
Gr. Kolchikón
Gr. Κολχικόν
H. Őszi kikerics
P. Zimowit jesienny
T. Sonbahar çiğdemi; Güzçiğdemi

211. Collinsonia canadensis
E. Stone Root; Horsebalm
F. Baume de cheval
G. Collinsonie
S. Hästmynta
It. Collinsonia
Gr. Kollinsónia i
   kanadhikí
Gr. Κολλινσόνια η καναδική
H. Kurtaszirom
T. İrmikökü

212. Colutea arborescens
E. Bladder Senna
F. Baguenaud; Faux Séné
G. Blasenkraut
S. Blåsärt
Sp. Espantalobos
It. Colutea; Vescicaria
Gr. Foúska
Gr. Φούσκα
H. Pukkantó dudafűrt;
   Varjúköröm
P. Moszenki
T. Yalan sinemeki

213. Commiphora molmol/
Myrrha
E. Myrrh
F. Myrrhe
G. Myrrhe
S. Myrra
Sp. Mirra
It. Mirra
Gr. Smýrna
Gr. Σμύρνα
H. Mirha
P. Mirra
T. Mer; Mır; Murr

214. Commiphora
opobalsamum
E. Balsam of Gilead
F. Baume de Gilead; Baume de la
   Mecque
G. Mekkabalsam; Opobalsam
S. Meckabalsamträd
Sp. Bilsamo
It. Balsamo di Palestina; Balsamo
   di Mecca
Gr. Válsamo Mékkas
Gr. Βάλσαμο Μέκκας
H. Mekkai balzsamfa
P. Balsam Mekka
T. Belesen ağ. Mekke pelsengi ağ

215. Conium maculatum
E. Hemlock
F. Grande ciguë
G. Schierling
S. Myrkkykatko
Sp. Cicuta
It. Cicuta maggiore
Gr. Kónion
Gr. Κώνειον
H. Bürök
P. Szczwół
T. Baldıran; Sukıran; Büyük
   baldıran

216. Consolida regalis
E. Wild Larkspur; Wild
   Delphinium
F. Dauphinelle des champs; Pied
   d'alouette
G. Feld Rittersporn; Acker
   Rittersporn
S. Riddarsporre
Sp. Espuela silvestre

It. Speronella consolida; Erba
   cornetta
Gr. Dhelphínio
Gr. Δελφίνιο
H. Vad sarkantyúvirág
P. Sroczka; Ostróżeczka
T. Horozkuyruğu; Keyiflice otu

217. Convallaria majalis
E. Lily-of-the-Valley
F. Muguet des bois
G. Maiglöckchen
S. Liljekonvalj
Sp. Lirio de los valles; Campanas
   de mayo
It. Mughetto
Gr. Mayátikos krínos
Gr. Μαγιάτικος κρίνος
H. Gyöngyvirág
P. Konwalia majus
T. Büyük inci çiç; Mayıs çiç.

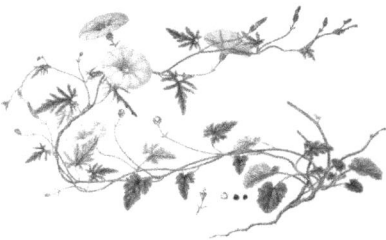

218. Convolvulus arvensis
E. Field Bindweed; Cornbine
F. Liseron des champs
G. Ackerwinde
S. Åker vinda
Sp. Altabaquillo; Campanilla
It. Convolvolo; Vilucchio comune
Gr. Perikokládha
Gr. Περικοκλάδα

H. Folyóka,földi
P. Powój polny
T. Çadır çiç.; Tarla sarmaşığı

219. Convolvulus sepium
E. Hedge Bindweed; Greater
   Bindweed
F. Liseron des haies
G. Zaunwinde
S. Snårvinda
Sp. Correhuela mayor
It. Convolvolo bianco
Gr. Kalísteghi perikokládha
Gr. Καλύστεγη περικοκλάδα
H. Folyóka, sövény
P. Powój
T. Çit sarmaşığı

220. Conyza canadensis→
Erigeron canadensis

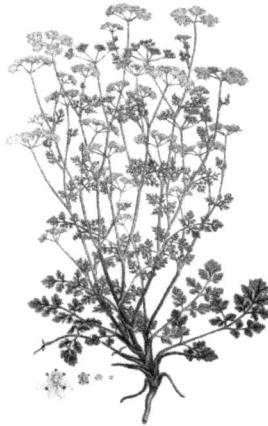

221. Coriandrum sativum
E. Coriander
F. Coriandre
G. Koriander

S. Koriander
Sp. Cilantro
It. Coriandola
Gr. Koríandhron
Gr. Κοϱίανδϱον
H. Koriander
P. Koryander; Kolendra
T. Kişniş otu

222. Coronilla varia
E. Crown Vetch
F. Coronille Bigarée
G. Kronwicke
S. Rosenkronill
Sp. Coronilla morada; Arvejilla
   morada
It. Veccierina; Coronilla
Gr. Kavelerú
Gr. Καβελεϱού
H. Tarka koronafürt
P. Cieciorka pstra
T. Renkli burçak; Körigen

223. Corydalis bulbosa
E. Purple Corydalis
F. Corydale creuse; Corydale
   bulbeuse
G. Hohler Lerchensporn
S. Stor nunneört
Sp. Coridal
It. Colombina solida
Gr. Korydhalís
Gr. Κοϱυδαλίς
P. Kokorycz pełna
T. Soğanlı kazgagası

224. Coryllus avellana
E. Hazelnut
F. Noisette

G. Haselnuss
S. Hassel
Sp. Avellana; Allano
It. Nocciolo
Gr. Foudoúki
Gr. Φουντούκι
H. Mogyoró
P. Leszczyna
T. Fındık

225. Crambe maritima
E. Sea Kale
F. Chou marin; Crambe
G. Meerkohl; Seekohl
S. Strandkål
Sp. Col maritime; Col marina
It. Cavolo di mare
Gr. Krámvi tis paralías
Gr. Κϱάμβη της παϱαλίας
H. Tengeri káposzta
P. Morska kapusta; Modrak
   morski
T. Deniz lahanası

226. Crataegus oxycantha
E. Hawthorn
F. Aubépine
G. Weissdorn
S. Trubbhagtorn
Sp. Espino blanco
It. Biancospino
Gr. Krátegos; Bourboutzeliá;
   Trikokiá
Gr. Κϱάταιγος·
   Μπουϱμπουτζελιά·
   Τϱικοκιά
H. Galagonya
P. Głóg dwuszyjkowy; Bodłak
T. Beyaz diken; Alıç; Edren

227. *Crithmum maritimum*
E. Rock Samphire
F. Christe-marin; Fenouil marin
G. Meerfenchel
S. Saltmärke
Sp. Hinojo marino
It. Finocchio marina
Gr. Almiriá; Almirikiá; Kritámi
Gr. Αλμιριά˙ Αλμιρικιά˙
   Κριτάμι
H. Tengeri kömény
P. Kowniatki; Babia sól
T. Deniz teresi; Kaya koroğu

228. *Crocus sativus*
E. Saffron Crocus
F. Safran cultivé
G. Safran-Krokus
S. Saffran
Sp. Azafrán
It. Zafferano
Gr. Krókos; Zaphorá
Gr. Κρόκος˙ Ζαφορά
H. Sáfrány
P. Szafran
T. Zafran

229. *Croton eluteria*
E. Cascarilla
F. Cascarille; Bois de crocodile
G. Kaskarilla
S. Kaskarilla
Sp. Cascarilla
It. Cascarilla; Legno coccodrillo
Gr. Kaskarílla
Gr. Κασκαρίλλα
H. Kaszkarilla
P. Kaskarylla
T. Amber kabuğu

230. *Croton lecheri*
E. Dragon"s Blood; Croton
F. Croton
G. Kroton
S. Kroton
Sp. Sangre de drago
It. Croton
Gr. Psevdhokróton o dhrákon
Gr. Ψευδοκρότων ο δράκων
P. Kroton smoczy
T. Kroton; Ejderhanın kanı

231. *Croton tiglium*
E. Purging Croton
F. Croton révulsif
G. Krotonölbaum; Purgierbaum
S. Krotonoljeträd
Sp. Croton
It. Croton purgante
Gr. Psevdhokroton o tiglios
Gr. Ψσευδοκρότων ο τίγλιος
H. Tejfű kroton
P. Kroton przeczyszczajy
T. Kroton 1

232. *Cryptogramma crispa*
E. Rockbreak; Parsley Fern
F. Cryptogramme; Allosore crépu
G. Rollfarn; Petersilienfarn
S. Krusbräken
It. Felcetta crispa
Gr. Kryptógramma
Gr. Κρυπτόγραμμα
H. Bodorpáfrány
P. Zmienka górska
T. Sakli eğrelti

233. *Cucumis sativa*
E. Cucumber

F. Concombre; Cornichon
G. Gurke
S. Gurka
Sp. Pepino; Cocombro
It. Cetriolo
Gr. Agoúri
Gr. Αγγούρι
H. Uborka
P. Ogórek
T. Hıyar fidani

234. Cucurbita pepo
E. Marrow; Pumpkin; Squash
F. Courge; Citrouille; Potiron;
   Courgette
G. Kürbis
S. Pumpa
Sp. Calabacera; Calabaza;
   Ahuyama
It. Zucca; Zucchini
Gr. Kolokíthi
Gr. Κολοκύθι
H. Tök
P. Kabaczek; Dynia
T. Adi küçük; Kabak

235. Cuminum cyminum
E. Cumin
F. Cumin
G. Kreuzkümmel
S. Kummin
Sp. Comino
It. Cumino
Gr. Kíminon
Gr. Κύμινον
H. Római kömény
P. Kmin
T. Kimyon

236. Cupressus sempervirens
E. Cypress
F. Cyprès
G. Zypresse
S. Cypress
Sp. Ciprés
It. Cipresso
Gr. Kiparíssi
Gr. Κυπαρίσσι
H. Ciprus
P. Cyprys
T. Akdeniz servisi

237. Curcuma longa
E. Turmeric
F. Safran des Indes; Curcuma
G. Gelbwurzel; Kurkuma
S. Gurkmeja
Sp. Batatilla; Curcuma larga
It. Curcuma; Zafferano dell' India
Gr. Kourkoúmas; Chrisóriza
Gr. Κουρκούμας· Χρυσόριζα
H. Kurkuma
P. Kurkuma długa
T. Kurkum; Hint zafran

238. Cuscuta europaea
E. Dodder
F. Grande cuscute
G. Hopfenseide; Kleeseide
S. Nässelsnärja
Sp. Cuscuta europea; Cabellos de
   Venus
It. Cuscuta europea
Gr. Kuskoúti; Neraidhónima
Gr. Κουσκούτη· Νεραϊδόνημα
H. Aranka; Fünyüg;
   Aranyfonalfű

P. Kanianka
T. Küsküt otu

239. *Cyamopsis tetragonolobus*
E. Guar
F. Guar
G. Guar
S. Guarböna
Sp. Guar
It. Guar
Gr. Goúar
Gr. Γκουάρ
H. Csomósbab; Guar
P. Guar

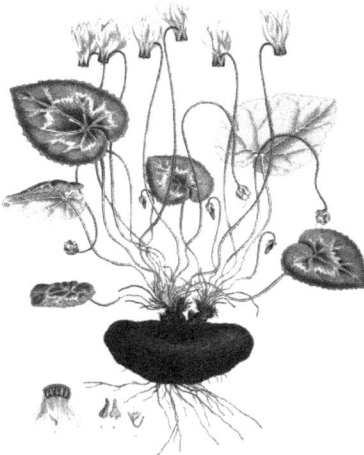

Cyclamen europeum

240. *Cyclamen europeum*
E. Cyclamen
F. Cyclamen
G. Alpenveilchen
S. Cyklamen
Sp. Ciclamen
It. Ciclamino
Gr. Kyklámino
Gr. Κυκλάμινο

H. Ciklámen
P. Gduła; Cyklamen dziki
T. Buhurumeryem (siklamen)

241. *Cydonia oblonga*
E. Quince
F. Coing
G. Quitte
S. Kvitten
Sp. Membrillero
It. Cotogna
Gr. Kydhóni
Gr. Κυδώνι
H. Birsalma
P. Pigwa
T. Ayva ağ.

242. *Cymbopogen citratus*
E. Lemongrass
F. Citronelle; Sereh
G. Zitronengras
S. Citrongräs
Sp. Hierba limon
It. Citronella; Barboncino limone
Gr. Lemonóhorto
Gr. Λεμονόχορτο
H. Fenyerfű
P. Palczatka cytrynowa
T. Limon otu

243. *Cymbopogen martinii*
E. Palmarosa
F. Palmarosa
G. Palmarosa
S. Palmrosgräs
Sp. Palmarosa
It. Palmarosa
Gr. Palmarósa
Gr. Παλμαρόζα
H. Pálmarózsafű

244. *Cynara scolymus*
E. Artichoke
F. Artichaut
G. Artischocke
S. Krönartskocka
Sp. Alcachofa
It. Carciofo
Gr. Anginára
Gr. Αγκινάρα
H. Articsóka
P. Karczoch
T. Enginar

245. *Cynoglossum officinale*
E. Hound's tongue
F. Cynoglosse
G. Hundszunge
S. Hundtunga
Sp. Besnuela; Cinoglosa
It. Lingua di cane; Cinoglossa
Gr. Kynóglossa; Skilóglossa
Gr. Κοινόγλωσσα·
    Σκυλόγλωσσα
H. Ebnyelvfű
P. Psi język; Ostrzeń pospolity
T. Köpek dili; Göz pıtrğı

246. *Cyperus papyrus*
E. Papyrus
F. Papyrus
G. Papyrusgras
S. Papyrus
Sp. Papiro
It. Papiro
Gr. Pápiros
Gr. Πάπυρος
H. Papiruszkáka
P. Papirus

T. Papirüs

247. *Cyperus rotundus*
E. Nutgrass; Sedge Root
F. Souchet rond
G. Nussegge; Nussgras
S. Nötag
Sp. Coquito; Coyolillo
It. Cipro orientale, Cipero
Gr. Kýpiros i strogilórizos
Gr. Κύπιρος η στρογγυλόριζος
H. Szíriai palka
P. Cybora
T. Topalak

248. *Cyprepedium pubescens*
E. Lady's Slipper
F. Sabot de Venus
G. Frauenschuh
S. Guckoska
Sp. Zapatito de dama
It. Scarpetta di Venere
Gr. Kipripódhion
Gr. Κυπριπόδιον
H. Vénusz cipellője; Rigópohár
P. Obuwik; Trzewiczlik
T. Hanım pabuç otu

249. *Cytisus scoparius*
E. Broom
F. Cytise; Genêt à balais
G. Besenginster
S. Harris
Sp. Heniesta de escobaso
It. Citiso scorpario; Ginistra dei
    carboni
Gr. Kítisos; Ammóhorta
Gr. Κύτισος; Αμμόχορτο

H. Seprözanót
P. Żarnowiec miolasty
T. Katır çiç. Katır tırnağı

250. *Daphne gnidium*
E. Garou Bush; Spurge Flax
F. Garou; Sainbois
G. Herbstseidelbast
Sp. Torvisco; Bufalaga;
   Matapolla
It. Gnidio; Erba corsa
Gr. Thimélea; Knídhion
Gr. Θημέλεα· Κνίδιον
H. Boroszlán
P. Wawarzynek
T. Beyneb fıdanı

251. *Daphne mezereon*
E. Mezereon
F. Daphné mézéréon;
   Bois-gentil
G. Seidelbast; Kellerhals
S. Tibast
Sp. Mecereo; Laureola hembra;
   Leño gentil
It. Dafne mezereo
Gr. Mezairéon; Holokoúki
Gr. Μεζαιρέον· Χολοκούκι
H. Farkas boroszlán
P. Wawrzynek wilczełyko
T. Mezeryon

252. *Datura stramonium*
E. Thornapple; Datura;
   Jimsonweed
F. Stramoine; Pomme épineuse;
   Datura
G. Stechapfel; Tollkraut

S. Spikklubba
Sp. Datura; Estramonia
It. Stramonia; Indormia
Gr. Datúra; Pordhóhorto;
   Tatoúlas
Gr. Ντατούρα· Πορδόχορτο·
   Τατούλας
H. Csattanó maszlag
P. Bieluń dziędzierzawa
T. Tatula; Şeytan elmasi

253. *Daucus carota*
E. Wild Carrot
F. Carotte sauvage
G. Möhre, wilde
S. Vild morot
Sp. Zanahoria silvestre
It. Carota selvatica
Gr. Ághrio karóto
Gr. Άγριο καρότο
H. Vad sárgarépa; Vad
   murok
P. Marchew zwyczajna
T. Yabani havuç

254. *Daucus carota sativus*
E. Carrot
F. Carotte
G. Karotte; Möhre;
   Mohrrübe
S. Morot
Sp. Zanahoria
It. Carota
Gr. Karóto
Gr. Καρότο
H. Sárgarépa
P. Marchew
T. Havuç

255. *Delphinium consolida*→
Consolida regalis

256. *Dianthus caryophyllus*
E. Carnation Pink
F. Œillet
G. Gartennelke
S. Trägårdsnejlika
Sp. Clavel
It. Garofano
Gr. Garífalo
Gr. Γαρύφαλο
H. Kerti szegfű
P. Goździk ogrodowy
T. Karanfil çiç.

257. *Digitalis lanata*
E. Grecian Foxglove; Woolly
    Foxglove
F. Digitale laineuse
G. Wolliger Fingerhut
S. Grekisk fingerborgsblomma
Sp. Dedalera griega.
It. Digitale greca
Gr. Didzitális i eriódhis;
    Dhaktilítis
Gr. Ντιτζιτάλις η εριόδης·
    Δακτυλίτις
H. Gyapjas gyűszűvirág
P. Naparstica wełnista
T. Yüksükotu yünlü

258. *Digitalis lutea*
E. Yellow Foxglove
F. Digitale jaune
G. Gelber Fingerhut
S. Liten fingerborgsblomma
Sp. Digital amarilla; Dedalera
    amarilla

It. Digitale gialla
Gr. Didzitális i kítrini; Dhaktilítis
Gr. Ντιτζιτάλις η κίτρινη·
    Δακτυλίτις
H. Sárga gyűszűvirág
P. Napartnica żólta
T. Yüksükotu şarı

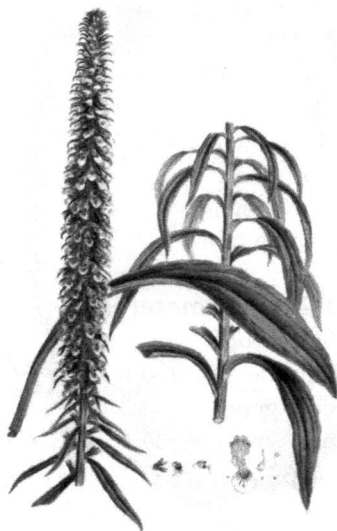

259. *Digitalis purpurea*
E. Common Foxglove
F. Digitale pourpre
G. Roter Fingerhut
S. Fingerborgsblomma
Sp. Digital; Azalda; Catechos
It. Digitale
Gr. Didzitális i porphirí;
    Dhaktilítis
Gr. Ντιτζιτάλις η πορφυρή·
    Δακτυλίτις
H. Gyűszűvirág
P. Naparstnica pospolita
T. Yüsükotu kırmızı

260. *Dioscorea villosa*
E. Wild Yam; Colic Root
F. Igname sauvage; Dioscorée;
Yam
G. Wilde Yamwurzel
S. Vildjams
Sp. Name; Dioscorea
It. Dioscorea selvatica
Gr. Yam.; Dhioskoréa
Gr. Γιάμ˙ Διοσκορέα
H. Ideggyökér
P. Pochrzyn
T. Yabani ığnam

261. *Dipsacus fullonum*
E. Teasel
F. Cardère sauvage; Cardère à
foulon
G. Wilde Karde; Rauhkarde
S. Kardvädd; Kardtistel
Sp. Cardencha
It. Scardaccione
Gr. Dhípsakos; Nerágatho
Gr. Δίψακος˙ Νεράγκαθο
H. Takács mácsonya
P. Szczeć pospolita
T. Çoban tarağı; Fescitarağı

262. *Dipteryx odorata*
E. Tonka Bean
F. Coumaron; Tonka fève
G. Tonkabohnen
S. Tonkaböna
Sp. Tonga; Yape
It. Fava Tonka
Gr. Fáva Tónka
Gr. Φάβα Τόνκα
H. Tonka bab

P. Tonka; Tonka bób
T. Tonka tohumu

263. *Dodonea viscosa*
E. Sticky Hop Bush
F. Bois de reinette;
Mangle-oseille
G. Sandolive; Felsenweide
S. Trevingebuske
Sp. Hayuela; Chanamo
I. Dodonea viscosa
Gr. Dhodhonea i ixódhis
Gr. Δωδωναία η ιξώδης
H. Enyves sziklafű
P. Oskrzydla
T. Dodenya

264. *Dorema ammoniacum*
E. Ammoniac Gum
F. Doreme ammoniac
G. Ammoniak
S. Dorema
Sp. Dorema; Amoniaco goma
It. Gomma Ammoniaco
Gr. Ammoníakon kommi
Gr. Αμμονίακον κόμμι
H. Ammóniák-gumi
P. Amoniaczek gumodajny
T. Uşak ağ; Çadır uşağı

265. *Dorestenia contrayerva*
E. Contrayerba
F. Contrayerva
G. Widergift
S. Besoarrot
Sp. Contrayerba
It. Contraierva
H. Bezoárgyökér

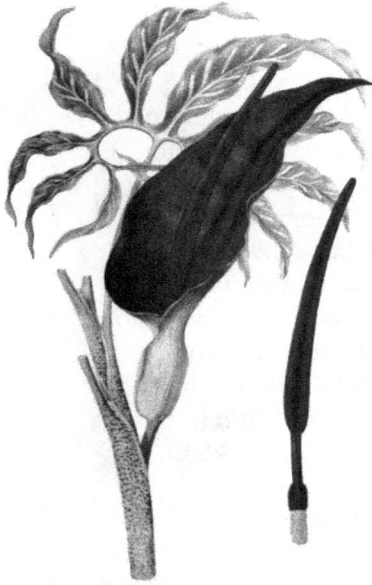

266. Dracunculus vulgaris
E. Dragon-Arum
F. Draconcule vulgaire
G. Drachenwurz
S. Drakkalla
Sp. Culebrina; Dragonera
   atrapa-mosca
It. Erba serpentaria; Dragontea
Gr. Dhrakondiá
Gr. Δρακοντιά
H. Sárkány-kontyvirág
P. Torun
T. Yilanbıçağı

267. Drimys winteri
E. Winter's Bark
F. Écorce de Winter; Canelle de
   Magallen
G. Winterrinden
S. Magellansk kanelträd
Sp. Canelo de paramo

It. Corteccio di Winter
Gr. Dhrímys o Wintérios
Gr. Δρίμυς ο Ουιντέριος
H. Magellán-fahéjcserje
P. Zacierp
T. Kışın kabuğu ağacı

268. Drosera rotundifolia
E. Sundew; Dewplant
F. Rosée du soleil; Drosera
G. Sonnenthau
S. Rundsileshår
Sp. Drósera; Rosa solis; Hierba
   de la gota
It. Drosera; Erba da fottosi
Gr. Dhroserá; Dhiónaia
Gr. Δροσερά· Διοναία
H. Harmatfű
P. Rosiczka; Rośnik
T. Çih otu; Güneş gülü

269. Dryas octopetala
E. Mountain Avens
F. Chénette; Dryas à huit petals
G. Silberwurz
S. Fjällsippa
Sp. Driada
It. Camedrio; Erba del cervo
Gr. Dhrías i ochtapétali
Gr. Δρίας η οκταπέταλη
H. Driasz; Magcsákó
P. Sylinic; Dębik
   ośmopłatkowy
T. Dağ gülü

270. Dryopteris felix-mas
E. Male Fern
F. Fougère male; Néphrode;
   Aspidie

G. Wurmfarn; Waldfarn;
Federfarn
S. Träjon
Sp. Helecho macho; Fayera
It. Felce maschio
Gr. Arenópteris; Ftéra
Gr. Αρενόπτερις· Φτέρα
H. Páfrány
P. Narecznica samcza
T. Erkek eğrelti

271. Duboisia myroporoides
E. Corkwood
F. Duboisie myopore
G. Korkholz
S. Duboisia
Sp. Pituri; Alcomoque
It. Duboisia
Gr. Dhuboisia
Gr. Δουμπόισια
H. Amerikai parafa
T. Avustralya mantar ağ.

272. Ecballium elaterium
E. Squirting Cucumber
F. Mormordique; Cornichon
sauvage
G. Spritzgurke
S. Springgurka
Sp. Pepinillo del diablo
It. Sputaveleno; Eletaria;
Cocomero asinino
Gr. Pikrangouriá
Gr. Πικραγγουριά
H. Közönséges magrugó
P. Tryskowiec lekarski
T. Eşek hıyarı; Acı kavun

273. Echinacea angustifolium
E. Echinacea; Cone Flower

F. Échinacée
G. Echinacea; Sonnenhut
S. Rudbeckia; Echinacea
Sp. Echinacea
It. Echinacea
Gr. Ekinátsia; Rudbékia
Gr. Εκινάτσια· Ρουντμπέκια
H. Ekinászia
P. Czesłota; Jeżówka
T. Ekinezya

274. Echinacea purpurea→
Echinacea angustifolium

275. Echium vulgare
E. Viper's Bugloss
F. Vipérine; Langue d'oie
G. Blauer Heinrich;
Natternkopf
S. Båeld
Sp. Viborera morada
It. Viperina; Echio comune
Gr. Voydhóglossa
Gr. Βοϊδόγλωσσα
H. Terjöke kígyószisz
P. Żmijowiec
T. Havacına otu

276. Eleutherococus senticosa
E. Siberian Ginseng;
Eleutherococus
F. Eleuthérocoque
G. Taigawurzel
S. Rysk rot
Sp. Eleuterococo
It. Eleuterococcos
Gr. Eleutherókokos
Gr. Ελευθερόκοκος
H. Tajgagyökér; Szibériai
ginszeng

P. Żeń-szeń syberyjsk
T. Sibirya ginsengi

277. Elletaria cardamomum
E. Cardamom
F. Cardamone
G. Kardamonpflanze
S. Kardemmuma
Sp. Cardamomos
It. Cardamomo
Gr. Kárdhamo
Gr. Κάρδαμο
H. Malabár kardamomom
P. Kardamon
T. Küçük kakule

278. Ephedra distachya
E. Ephedra; Joint Pine
F. Éphédre; Uvette
G. Gewöhnliches Meerträubel
S. Efedra
Sp. Efedra
It. Efedra
Gr. Ephédra; Kondhilóhorto
Gr. Εφέδρα· Κονδυλόχορτο
H. Csikófark
P. Prześl; Efedra
T. Deniz üzümü; Efedra

279. Epilobium angustifolium
E. Rose-Bay-Willow-Herb;
  Fireweed
F. Épilobe; Saulaie
G. Waldweidenröschen
S. Dunrav mjölkört
Sp. Epilobio
It. Epilobo; Lauro roseo
Gr. Epilóbio to stenófilo
Gr. Επιλόμπιο το στενόφυλλο

H. Füzike
P. Wierzbówka kiprzyca
T. Mukaddes defne; Yakı otu

280. Equisitum arvense
E. Horsetail
F. Prèle des champs;
  Queue-de-chat
G. Schachtelhalm, acker
S. Åkerfräken; Rövrumpa
Sp. Cola de caballo; Equisito
It. Coda Cavallino; Equiseto
Gr. Equizéto; Polykómbi;
  Polytríchi
Gr. Εκουιζέτο·
  Πολυκόμπι·Πολυτρίχι
H. Zsúrló
P. Strzępka; Skrzyp
T. At kuyruğı

281. Erigeron canadensis
E. Canadian Fleabane;
  Horseweed
F. Érigéron du Canada
G. Kanadische Berufkraut
S. Kanadabinka
Sp. Erigero; Avoadinha
It. Saeppola; Impia
Gr. Erígheron
Gr. Ερίγερον
H. Betyárkóró
P. Przmiotno kanadyjskie
T. Çakal otu; Kanada şifa otu

282. Eriobotrya japonica
E. Loquat
F. Bibacier; Néflier du Japon
G. Japanische Wollmispel
S. Japansk mispel

Sp. Nispero
It. Nespole
Gr. Mousmoula
Gr. Μούσμουλο
H. Japán naspolya
P. Nieśplik japónski
T. Yeni dünya ağ.

283. *Eriodictyon glutinosum*
E. Yerba Santa
F. Eriodyction
G. Gemeiner Reiherschnabel
S. Yerba santa
Sp. Yerba Santa
It. Erba Santa; Eriodicto
Gr. Eriódhikto
Gr. Εριόδικτο

284. *Erodium cicutarium*
E. Storksbill; common
F. Bec de grue
G. Storchenschnabel
S. Skatnäva
Sp. Alfilerillo de pastor;
    Ciguenas; Pico de grulla
It. Rostra di gru; Cicutaria
Gr. Kalógheros; Eródhion
Gr. Καλόγερος· Ερώδιον
H. Bürökgémorr
P. Iglica pospolita
T. Dönbabaotu; Çobanığnesi

285. *Eryngium campestre*
E. Field Eryngo
F. Panicaut; Chardon
    Roland
G. Feld Mannstreu
S. Martorn
Sp. Cardo corredor

It. Calcatreppolo campestre;
    Bocca di cucio
Gr. Erýghio; Moskágatho
Gr. Ερύγιο· Μοσκάγκαθο
H. Iringó
P. Mikolajek polny; Latawiec
T. Ibrahim dikeni; Buğa dikeni

286. *Eryngium maritimum*
E. Sea Holly
F. Panicaut de mer
G. Stranddistel; Meer-Mannstreu
S. Havsmartorn; Kostertistel
Sp. Eringio marítimo
It. Calcatreppolo marittimo;
    Cardio stellario
Gr. Galanóhorto; Erýghion to
    parálion
Gr. Γαλανόχορτο· Ερύγιον το
    παράλοιον
H. Tengeri iringó
P. Mikołajek nadmorski
T. Büyük boğa dikeni; Yılan dikeni

287. *Erythraea centaurium*→
Centranthus ruber

288. *Erythroxylum coca*
E. Coca; Cocaine
F. Coca; Cocaïne
G. Koka
S. Koka
Sp. Coca
It. Coca
Gr. Kóka
Gr. Κόκα
H. Kókacserje
P. Koka
T. Koka

289. *Eschscholtzia californica*
E. Californian Poppy
F. Pavot de Californie;
   Eschscholtzia
G. Kalifornischer Mohn
S. Sömntuta
Sp. Amapola de California
It. Escolzia di California
Gr. Eschóltsia i Kaliforniakí
Gr. Εσχόλτσια η
   Καλιφορνιακή
H. Kaliforniai mák
P. Pozłotka kalifornijska
T. Acem lalesi; Kaliforniya
   haşhaşı

290. *Eucalyptus spp.*
E. Eucalyptus
F. Eucalyptus
G. Eukalyptus
S. Eukalyptus
Sp. Eucalipto
It. Eucalipto
Gr. Efkályptos
Gr. Ευκάλυπτος
H. Eukaliptusz
P. Eukaliptus
T. Sıtma ağ; Okaliptüs

291. *Eugenia caryophyllata*
E. Clove
F. Girofle
G. Nelke
S. Kryddnejlikträd
Sp. Clavos; Jerofle
It. Garofano, chiodo di
Gr Garífalo
Gr. Γαρύφαλο
H. Szegfűszeg
P. Pierna

T. Bahar karanfil

292. *Euonymus europaeus*
E. Spindle
F. Fusain; Bonnet de prêtre
G. Spindelstrauch; Pfaffenhütchen
S. Benved
Sp. Evónimo; Aliso negro
It. Fusaria comune; Berretta da
   prete
Gr. Evónymos; Aspróxilo
Gr. Ευόνυμος˙ Ασπρόξυλο
Ar. Ariqîyat er raheb
Ar. عرقية الراهب
H. Kecskerágó
P. Trzmielina europejska
T. İğcik ağacı

293. *Eupatorium cannabinum*
E. Hemp Agrimony
F. Eupatoire chanvrine
G. Wasserdost
S. Hampflockel
Sp. Eupatorio de agua; Eriketa
It. Canapa acquatica; Eupatorio
Gr. Evpatórion to kannavinón
Gr. Ευπατόριον το καναβινόν
H. Sédkender
P. Sadziec konopiasty
T. Koyun butrağı; Yaban keteni

294. *Eupatorium perfoliatum*
E. Boneset; Feverwort
F. Herbe à fièvre; Herbe à souder
G. Durchwaschener Wasserhanf
S. Vattenhampa
Sp. Eupatoria
I. Canapa acquatica americana
Gr. Evpatório to dhiáfilo
Gr. Ευπατόριο το διάφυλλο

H. Amerikai lázgyöker
T. Amerikan su keneveri

295. Eupatorium purpureum
E. Gravel Root; Hempweed; Joe
   Pye Weed
F. Eupatoire pourpre
G. Kunigundenkraut
S. Rosenflockel
Sp. Eupatorio
It. Canapa purpurea
Gr. Evpatório to porfyró
Gr. Ευπατόριο το πορφυρό
H. Sédkender
P. Upatrek
T. Grip otu; Kirmizi keneviri

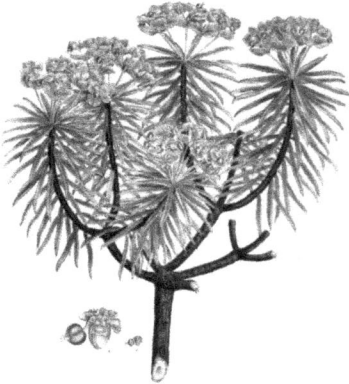

Euphorbia dendroides.

296. Euphorbia hirta
E. Garden Spurge; Asthma Weed
F. Épurge; Euphorbe pilulifère
G. Wolfsmilch
S. Pillertörel
Sp. Golondrina
It. Euforbia pilulifera
Gr. Evfórvion; Galatsídha
Gr. Εὐφόρβιον· Γαλατσίδα

H. Kutyatej
P. Wilczomlecz
T. Hint sütleğen otu

297. Euphorbia peplis
E. Purple Spurge
F. Euphorbe pêplis
G. Rote Wolfsmilch
S. Rävtörel
Sp. Esula redonda
It. Euforbia minore
Gr. Evfórvia péplis
Gr. Ευφόρβια πέπλις
H. Farkas kutyatej
P. Wilczomlecz ogrodowy
T. Kıyı sütleğeni

298. Euphrasia officinale
E. Eyebright
F. Casse-lunettes
G. Augentröst
S. Finnögontröst
Sp. Luminaria; Eufrasia
It. Evfrasia
Gr. Evfrásia
Gr. Ευφράσια
H. Szemvidítófű
P. Świetlik
T. Göz otu; Ufrazia otu

299. Fagopyrum esculentum
E. Buckwheat
F. Sarrasin; Blé noir
G. Buchenweizen; Heikedorn
S. Bovete
Sp. Alforojon; Trigoserracena
It. Grano saraceno
Gr. Triganósporos; Faghópyron
Gr. Τριγανόσπορος· Φαγόπυρον
H. Hajdina

P. Gryka; Hreczka; Tatarka
T. Kara buğday; Esmerbuğday

300. Fagus sylvatica
E. Beech
F. Hetre; Fayard
G. Buche
S. Bok
Sp. Haya
It. Faggio
Gr. Oxiá
Gr. Οξυά
H. Bükk
P. Buk
T. Kayın ağ.

301. Ferula asa-foetida
E. Asafoetida
F. Férule assafétide
G. Stinkasant
S. Dyvelsträck
Sp. Asafétida
It. Assafetida
Gr. Asifoétidha; Sýlphion
Gr. Ασιφαίτιδα΄ Σύλφιον
H. Ördöggyöker
P. Smrodliwa
T. Şeytan boku

302. Ferula gummosa
E. Galbanum
F. Galbanum
G. Rutenkraut
S. Galbanum
Sp. Galbano
It. Ferula
Gr. Feroula i kommiofóros
Gr. Φερούλα η κομμιοφόρος
H. Galbanum; Gumigyanta
P. Galbanum

T. Kesni; Kasnı otu

303. Ficus carica
E. Fig
F. Figue
G. Feige
S. Fikon
Sp. Higo; Brevo
It. Fico
Gr. Síko
Gr. Σύκο
H. Füge
P. Figowiec
T. İncir

304. Filipendula ulmaria
E. Meadowsweet
F. Reine des prés; Ulmaire
G. Mädesüss; Weisenkönigen
S. Äggräs
Sp. Reina de los prados; Ulmaria
It. Regina dei prati; Spirea
    ulmaria
Gr. Spiréa
Gr. Σπιρέα
H. Réti legyezőfű; Gyöngyvessző
P. Wiązówka błotna; Tawula;
    Ergeç sakali
T. Su Rezenesi; Keçi sakalı;
    Ergeç sakali

305. Filipendula vulgaris
E. Dropwort
F. Filipendule
G. Knolliges Mädsüss
S. Brudbröd
Sp. Filipendula
It. Olmaria peperina
Gr. Filipéndoula i kiní 305
Gr. Φιλιπέντουλα η κοινή 305

H. Koloncos legyezőfű
P. Wiązówka bulwkowata;
Ilmowna
T. Kandil çiçeği

306. *Foeniculum vulgare*
E. Fennel
F. Fenouil
G. Fenchel
S. Fänkål
Sp. Hinojo; Fenicula
It. Finocchio
Gr. Máratho
Gr. Μάραθο
H. Édes kömény
P. Fenkuł; Fankiel
T. Rezene; Razyane

307. *Fragaria vesca*
E. Strawberry
F. Fraise
G. Erdbeere
S. Smultron
Sp. Fresa
It. Fragola
Gr. Fráoula
Gr. Φράουλα
H. Eper
P. Truskawka
T. Çilek fıdanı

308. *Frangula alnus*
E. Alder Buckthorn;
F. Bourdaine
G. Faulbaum
S. Brakved
Sp. Araclán; Avellanillo
It. Frangola

Gr. Vourvouliá
Gr. Βουρβουλιά
H. Közönséges kutyabenge;
Kutyabenge; Fekete Égerfa
P. Kruszyna pospolita
T. Barut ağacı

309. *Fraxinus exelsior*
E. Ash
F. Fréne
G. Esche
S. Ask
Sp. Fresno
It. Frassino
Gr. Flamouriá
Gr. Φλαμουριά
H. Köris
P. Jesion
T. Diş budak; Asfur ağ

310. *Fraxinus ornus*
E. Manna Ash; Flake Manna
F. Frène à manne
G. Manna-Esche
S. Mannaask
Sp. Orno
It. Frassino manna; Orniella
Gr. Méleghos
Gr. Μέλεγος
H. Virágos kőrisfa
P. Jesion mannowy
T. Çiçekli dişbudak

311. *Fucus vesiculosus*
E. Bladder-wrack
F. Raisin de mer; Varech
vésiculeux
G. Blasentang; Meerblasentang

S. Blåstång
Sp. Fuco vejigoso; Alga feoficea
It. Quercia marina; Fucus
   vesiculosus
Gr. Fíkia thalásis
Gr. Φύκια θαλάσσης
H. Hólyagmoszat
P. Szuwar; Morszczyn
   pęcherzykowaty
T. Birtür deniz yosunu

312. Fumaria officinalis
E. Fumitory
F. Fumeterre
G. Erdrauch
S. Jordrök
Sp. Fumaria; Patomilla
It. Fumaria; Fecce
Gr. Kapnóhorto; Fumária
Gr. Καπνόχορτο· Φουμάρια
H. Füstike
P. Dymnica
T. Şahtere otu

313. Gagea lutea
E. Yellow Star of Bethlehem
F. Gagée des champs
G. Acker Gelbstern
S. Vårlök
Sp. Gagea de los campos
It. Cipollaccio
Gr. Ghagéa i kitriní
Gr. Γαγέα η κιτρινή
H. Ernyős madártej
P. Zloć
T. Sarı yıldız

314. Galanthus nivalis
E. Snowdrop
F. Perce-neige

G. Schneeglöckchen
S. Snödroppe
Sp. Flor de nieve
It. Bucaneve
Gr. Gálanthos
Gr. Γάλανθος
H. Hóvirág
P. Przebiśnieg; Śnieżyca
T. Kardelen

315. Galega officinalis
E. Goat's Rue; French Lilac
F. Rue de chèvre; Galéga
G. Geisseraute; Geissklee
S. Getruta
Sp. Ruda cabruna; Galega
It. Capraggine; Galega
Gr. Galéga
Gr. Γκαλέγκα
H. Kecskeruta
P. Rutwica
T. Keçi sedefi

316. Galeopsis tetrahit
E. Common Hemp-nettle
F. Ortie royale; Galéopsis
G. Hohlzahn; Sandhohlzahn
S. Pipdån
Sp. Ortiga real; Galeopsis
It. Canapaccia comune;
   Galeopside
Gr. Galeópsis
Gr. Γκαλεόπσις
H. Tarka kenderfű
P. Poziewnik
T. Yalan kenevır otu; Kedi başı

317. Galinsoga parviflora
E. Gallant Soldier; Joey Hooker
F. Galinsoga

G. Kleinblütiges Knopfkraut
S. Gängel
Sp. Soldado galante
It. Galinsoga
Gr. Ghalinsóga i vrachyanthís
Gr. Γαλινσόγα η
βραχυανθής
H. Kicsiny gombvirág
P. Żółtlica drobnokwiatowa
T. Beşpat çiçeği

318. Galipea officinalis
E. Angostura
F. Angostura; Cusparie
G. Angostura; Kuspa
S. Angostura
Sp. Angostura; Cuspa
It. Angostura; Cusparia
Gr. Angostúra
Gr. Ανγκοστούρα
H. Angosztura
P. Kusparia; Febrzystręt
T. Güzel kokulu bir ağaç

319. Galium aperine
E. Cleaver; Cliver; Goosegrass;
Sticky Willie
F. Gaillet grateron; Gaillet
acrochant; Grateoul
G. Klebkraut; Kletten-Labkraut
S. Snärjmåra
Sp. Amor de hortelano;
Azotalenguas
It. Attaccamani; Caglio asprello
Gr. Kolitsídha; Kavalariá
Gr. Κολιτσίδα· Καβαλαριά
H. Ragadós galaj
P. Przytulia czepna; Lepczyca
T. Dil kanatan; Çoban süzgeci;
Yapsikan otu

320. Galium verum
E. Lady's Bedstraw; Cheese
Rennet
F. Gaillet jaune; Gaillet
odorante
G. Labkraut
S. Gulmåra
Sp. Galio
It. Caglio giallo; Presuola
Gr. Ghálio
Gr. Γάλιο
H. Galaj
P. Przytulia właściwa
T. Boyalık; İlkbahar yoğurt otu;
Sarı yoğurt otu

321. Gaultheria procumbens
E. Wintergreen; Mountain Tea
F. Gautherie couchée; Thé du
Canada
G. Wintergrün; Scheinbeere
S. Tuvvaktelbär
Sp. Gaulteria
It. Tè di montagna
Gr. Gaultéria
Gr. Γκαουλτέρια
H. Gaulteria
P. Gaulteria rozesłana
T. Keklik üzümü

322. Gelidium amansii
E. Agar-Agar
F. Agar-Agar
G. Agar-Agar
Sp. Agar-Agar
It. Agar-Agar
Gr. Agár-Agár
Gr. Αγκάρ-Αγκάρ
H. Agar-Agar
P. Agar-Agar

T. Yogsun (kırmızı)

323. *Gelsemium sempervirens*
E. Yellow Jasmine
F. Gelsemie luisante
G. Gelber Jasmine
S. Giftjasmin
Sp. Gelsomina
It. Gelsemio
Gr. Yasemí kítrino
Gr. Γιασεμί κίτρινο
H. Sárga jázmin
P. Jaśmin żółty
T. Sarı yasemin

324. *Genista tintoria*
E. Dyers Greenwood; Dyer's Broom
F. Genêt des tinturiers
G. Fäberginster
S. Färgginst
Sp. Hiniesta de tintes; Retama de tintorero
It. Ginistrella
Gr. Afána; Yenísta i vafikí
Gr. Αφάνα· Γενίστα η βαφική
H. Festőrekettye
P. Janowiec barwierski; Drok gładki
T. Boyacı otu

325. *Gentiana lutea*
E. Yellow Gentian
F. Gentiane jaune; Grande gentiane
G. Gelber Enzian
S. Gullgentiana
Sp. Genciana
It. Genziana maggiore

Gr. Yentiána
Gr. Γεντιάνα
H. Tárnics; Gencian
P. Goryczka żółta
T. Güşad; Çentıyan otu

326. *Geranium maculatum*
E. Cranesbill
F. Geranium à rhizome
G. Kranichschnabel
S. Fläcknäva
Sp. Geranio silvestre
It. Geranio macchiato
Gr. Moscholáchano
Gr. Μοσχολάχανο
H. Gölyaorr
P. Bodziszek
T. Itır

327. *Geranium robertianum*
E. Herb Robert
F. Herbe à Robert
G. Robertgerme; Ruprechtskraut
S. Stinknäva
Sp. Hierba de San Roberto
It. Erba Roberto; Cicuta rossa
Gr. Yeránion to Rovertianó
Gr. Γεράνιον το Ροβερτιανό
H. Nehészagú gólyaorr
P. Bodziszek cuchnący
T. Turna ğağası

328. *Geum rivale*
E. Water Avens
F. Benoîte des ruisseaux
G. Bachnelkenwurz; Ufernelkwurz
S. Humleblomster
Sp. Orejuela de arroya

It. Benedetta; Ambretta d'acqua
Gr. Ghéo to parapotámio
Gr. Γέο το παραποτάμιο
H. Patakparti; Vízi gyömbér
P. Kuklik zwisły
T. Su karanfil otu; Su meryem otu

329. Geum urbanum
E. Wood Avens
F. Benoîte commun
G. Echte Nelkenwurz
S. Rejlikrot
Sp. Hierba de San Benito;
   Gariofilea
It. Cariofillata; Garofanaia
Gr. Ghéo to astikó
Gr. Γέο το αστικό
H. Erdei gyömbér
P. Kuklik pospolity
T. Karanfilköku

330. Gingko biloba
E. Gingko; Maidenhair Tree
F. Gingko
G. Gingko
S. Gingko
Sp. Gingko
It. Gingko
Gr. Gingko
Gr. Γκίνγκο
H. Páfrányfenyő.
P. Miłorząb dwuklapowy
T. Mabet ağ; Gingko

331. Glechoma hedera
E. Ground Ivy
F. Lierre terrestre
G. Gundermann; Gundelrebe
S. Jordreva
Sp. Hiedra terrestre

It. Edera terrestre
Gr. Hamókissos
Gr. Χαμόκισσος
H. Kerek repkény
P. Kurdybanek; Bluszczyk ziemny
T. Yer sarmaşığı

332. Globularia vulgaris
E. Common Globe Daisy;
   Common Globularia
F. Globulaire
G. Gewönliche Kugelblume
S. Bergsgrabba
Sp. Globularia mayor
It. Globularia; Margherita azzura
Gr. Globulária
Gr. Γκλομπουλάρια
H. Gubóvirág
P. Kulnik
T. Mavi ince çiç. Kurrevi

333. Glysine soya
E. Soya; Soya Bean
F. Soya; Pois Chinois
G. Sojabohne
S. Sojaböna
Sp. Soja; Soya
It. Soia; Soya
Gr. Sóya
Gr. Σόγια
H. Szójabab
P. Soja
T. Soya

334. Glycyrrhiza glabra
E. Liquorice
F. Réglisse
G. Süssholz
S. Lakritsros
Sp. Regaliz; Ozozura

It. Liquerizia
Gr. Ghlikóriza
Gr. Γλυκόριζα
H. Édesgyöker; Medvecukor
P. Lukrecja
T. Meyan kökü; Meyan otu;
    Biyan kökü

335. Gnaphilium dioica→
Antennaria dioica

336. Gnaphalium uliginosum
E. Cudweed; Cottonweed
F. Immortelle
G. Ruhrkraut
S. Sumpnoppa
Sp. Borrosa; Algodonosa
It. Canapicchie
Gr. Gnafálio to elóvio
Gr. Γναφάλιο το ελόβιο
H. Iszapgyopár
P. Szarota

337. Gossypium herbaceum
E. Cotton
F. Coton
G. Baumwolle
S. Bomull
Sp. Algodon
It. Cotone
Gr. Vamváki
Gr. Βαμβάκι
H. Gyapot; Pamut
P. Bawełna
T. Pambuk

338. Gratiola officinalis
E. Hedge Hyssop
F. Gratiole
G. Gnadenkraut

S. Jordgalla
Sp. Graciola
I. Graziola; Grazie Dei
Gr. Gratióla
Gr. Γρατιόλα
H. Csikorgófű; Csikorka
P. Konitrud; Trud
T. Fuara otu; Hüdaverdi otu

339. Grindelia camporum
E. Grindelia; Gumplant
F. Grindélie
G. Grindelkraut
S. Grindelior
Sp. Grindelia
It. Grindelia
Gr. Grindélia i pedhiní
Gr. Γκριντέλια η πεδινή
P. Doględawa
T. Grindelya

340. Guaiacum officinalis
E. Guaiacum; Lignum Vitae
F. Gayac
G. Guayac
S. Pockenholts
Sp. Guayaco; Guayacan
It. Guaiaco; Legno santo
Gr. Guayáko
Gr. Γουαϊάκο
H. Guajakfa; Pokfa
P. Gwajak
T. Guayak ağacı; Kutsal odun ağ;
    Peygamber ağ.

341. Hamamelis virginiana
E. Witch-Hazel
F. Hamamélis; Noisetier des
    sorcières
G. Virginischer Zauberstrauch

S. Amerikansk trollhassel
Sp. Hamamelis; Avellana de
   bruja
It. Amemelide; Hamamelis
Gr. Amamilís
Gr. Αμαμηλίς
H. Varázsfa; Bübájdio
P. Oczar; Czarnoksięzki
T. Güvercin; Cadi findigi;
   Hamamelis

**342. Harpagophytum
procumben**
E. Devil's Claw
F. Griffe-du-diable
G. Teufelskralle
S. Harpagoört
Sp. Harpago; Uña del diablo
It. Artiglio del diavolo
Gr. Arpaghóphyto
Gr. Αρπαγόφυτο
H. Ördögköröm
P. Czarci pazur
T. Şeytan pençesi

343. Hedera helix
E. Ivy
F. Lierre
G. Efeu
S. Murgröna
Sp. Hiedra; Yedra
It. Edera
Gr. Kissós
Gr. Κισσός
H. Repkény; Borostyán
P. Bluszcz
T. Sarmaşık; Duvarsarmaşığı

344. Helianthus annuus
E. Sunflower

F. Tournesol
G. Sonnenblume
S. Solros
Sp. Girasol
It. Girasole
Gr. Ilíanthos; Iliotrópio
Gr. Ηλίανθος; Ηλιοτρόπιο
H. Napraforgó
P. Słonecznik
T. Ay çiç. Gün çiç; Güne bakan

345. Helianthus tuberosus
E. Jerusalem Artichoke
F. Topinambour; Artichaut de
   Jèrusalem
G. Jerusalem Artischoke
S. Jordärtskocka
Sp. Pataca
It. Carciofo di Giudea;
   Topinambur
Gr. Psevthokolokásion; Ilíanthos
   o kondhylórizos
Gr. Ψευδοκολοκάσιον·
   Ηλίανθος ο κονδυλόριζος
H. Csicsóka
P. Topinambur; Słonecznik
   bulwiasty
T. Yıldız kökü; Yerelması

346. Helichrysum arenarium
E. Imortelle; Everlasting
F. Imortelle des sables
G. Sandstrohblume
S. Hedblomster
Sp. Perpetua; Siempreviva
It. Sempreviva; Immortale;
   Elicriso
Gr. Amáranto
Gr. Αμάραντο
H. Szalmagyopár

P. Kocanki; Suchotnik
T. Altınotu; Heremtaze; Ölmez çiçek

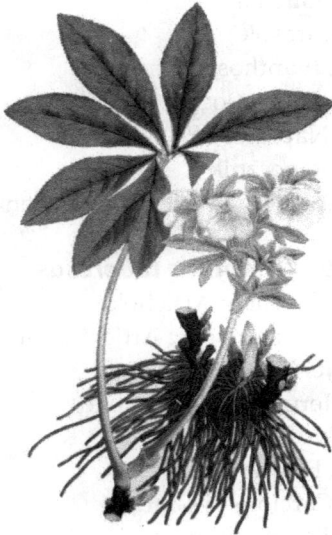

347. *Helleborus niger*
E. Black Hellebore; Christmas
   Rose
F. Hellèbore noir; Rose de noël
G. Schwarze Neiswurz;
   Christrose
S. Julros
Sp. Eléboro negro
It. Elleboro nero
Gr. Ellévoros; Skárfi
Gr. Ελλέβορος· Σκάρφη
H. Karácsony rózsa
P. Śnieżna róża; Ciemiernik
T. Noel gülü

348. *Helleborus viridis*
E. Green Hellebore; Bear's Foot
F. Hellèbore vert
G. Grüne Neiswurz
S. Grön julros

Sp. Eléboro verde
It. Elleboro verde
Gr. Ellévoros prásinos
Gr. Ελλέβορος πράσινος
H. Zöld hunyor; Zászpa
P. Ciemiernik zielony
T. Yeşil çöpleme

349. *Hepatica nobilis*
E. Liverwort; Liverleaf
F. Anémone hépatique
G. Leberblümchen; Märzblümchen
S. Blåsippa
Sp. Hepatica; Hepistica
It. Fegatella; Erba trinità; Epatica
Gr. Ipatikón evyenés
Gr. Ηπατικόν ευγενές
H. Májfű; Májvirág
P. Przylaszczka; Trojanek

350. *Heracleum sphondilium*
E. Cow parsnip; Hogweed; Keck
F. Grande berce; Patte d'ours
G. Weisen Bärenklau;
   Herkuleskraut
S. Björnloka
Sp. Belleraca; Ursina
It. Panace
Gr. Iráklio i sphondílio
Gr. Ηράκλειο το σφοντίλιο
H. Termetes medvetalp
P. Barszcz zwyczajny
T. Çayır tavşancılotu: Kamşam

351. *Herniaria glabra*
E. Rupturewort; Herniary
F. Herniaire; Herniole
G. Kahles Bruchkraut
S. Knytling
Sp. Herniaria; Arenal; Arenaria

It. Erniaria
Gr. Erniária
Gr. Ερνιάρια
H. Kopasz porcika
P. Źabie gronka; Połonicznik nagi
T. Kaşıkotu; Atyaran; Bozkırotu

352. Hibiscus abelmoschus
E. Muskseed
F. Ketmie odorante
G. Abelmoschus
S. Prakthibiskus
Sp. Ambretta
It. Ambretta; Grana moscata
Gr. Karkadé
Gr. Καρκαντέ
H. Ábelfű
P. Ketmia
T. Amber çiç.; Misk çiç.

353. Hibiscus esculentus
E. Okra; Lady Finger; Gumbo
F. Gombaud; Corne grecque; Okra
G. Okra
S. Okra
Sp. Quimbombó; Quinbombó
It. Ocra; Ibisco esculento
Gr. Bámya
Gr. Μπάμια
H. Gombó
P. Okra
T. Bamya

354. Hibiscus sabdariffa
E. Hibiscus; Roselle
F. Ketmie acide
G. Hibiskus; Karkade; Rosellahanf

S. Hibiscus
Sp. Hibisco; Rosella
It. Ibisco; Carcade; Esperide
Gr. Ivískos
Gr. Ιβίσκος
H. Hibiszkusz
P. Hibiskus; Poślubnik; Proświrnik
T. Hibiskus

355. Hieracium pilosella
E. Mouse-Eared Hawkweed
F. Piloselle; Oreille de souris
G. Mausohr Habichtskraut
S. Gråbfibbla
Sp. Vellosilla; Oreja de ratón
It. Pilosella
Gr. Ierátsio
Gr. Ιεράτσιο
H. Ezüstös hölgymál
P. Jaztrzębiec kosmaczek
T. Fare kulağı

356. Hippophaë rhamnoides
E. Sea Buckthorn
F. Argousier; Griset anglais
G. Sanddorn
S. Havtorn
Sp. Espino amarillo
It. Olivella spinosa
Gr. Ippophaés to ramnoidhés
Gr. Ιπποφαές το ραμνοϊδές
H. Ezüsttövis
P. Rokitnik zwyczajny
T. Yabani iğde ağ

357. Hordeum vulgare
E. Barley
F. Orge
G. Gerste

S. Korn
Sp. Cebada
It. Orzo
Gr. Krithári
Gr. Κριθάρι
H. Árpa
P. Fal; Jęczmień
T. Arpa

358. *Humulus lupulus*
E. Hops
F. Houblon
G. Hopfen
S. Humle
Sp. Lúpulo; Hombrecillo
It. Luppolo
Gr. Lisískos
Gr. Λυκίσκος
H. Komló
P. Chmiel
T. Himel; Şerbetçi otu

359. *Hydrangea arborescens*
E. Hydrangea
F. Hortensia
G. Hortensie
S. Hortensia
Sp. Hortensia
It. Ortensia
Gr. Ortánsia
Gr. Ορτάνσια
H. Hortenzia
P. Hortensja; Hidranga
T. Ortanca; Japon gülü

360. *Hydrastis canadensis*
E. Goldenseal; Yellowroot
F. Idraste du Canada; Sceau d'or
G. Kanadische Gelbwurzel;
    Kanadische Orangenwurzel

S. Hydrastis
Sp. Idraste; Raiz de oro
It. Idrastis; Sigillo d'oro
Gr. Idhrástis
Gr. Ηδράστις
H. Kanadai aranygyökér
P. Gorznik kanadyjski; Drobiałka
T. Altun mühür

361. *Hydrocotyle asiatica*
E. Gotu Kola; Indian Pennywort
F. Hydrocotyle; Centelle asiatique
G. Asiatisches Wassernabelkraut
S. India spikblad
Sp. Hidrocótile; Bero macho
It. Idrocotile; Centella asiatica
Gr. Gótou-kóla
Gr. Γκότου-κόλα
H. Ázsiai gázló
P. Wąkrot azjatycka
T. Gotu Kola

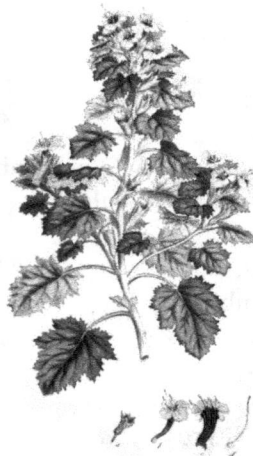

362. *Hyoscyamus niger*
E. Henbane
F. Jusquiame noir

G. Schwarzes Bilsenkraut
S. Bolmört
Sp. Beleño negro
It. Giusquiamo
Gr. Ioskyámos;
Dhemonariá
Gr. Υοσκύαμος· Δαιμοναριά
H. Beléndek
P. Lulek czarny; Lulka
T. Banotu; Bardakotu; Kara banotu

363. Hypericum perforatum
E. St John's Wort
F. Millpertuis perforé
G. Johanniskraut
S. Johannesört
Sp. Hiperico; Corazoncillo;
Hierba de San Juan
It. Iperico
Gr. Válsamo; Ipérikon;
Spathóhorto
Gr. Βάλσαμο· Υπέρικον·
Σπαθόχορτο
H. Tűzdeltlevelű; Orbáncfű
P. Świetojańskie ziele;
Dziurawiec
T. Sarı kantaron; Kantaron otu;
Binbir delik otu

364. Hyssopus officinalis
E. Hyssop
F. Hysope
G. Ysop; Essigkraut
S. Isop
Sp. Hisopo
It. Issopo
Gr. Issopos
Gr. Υσσωπος
H. Izsóp

P. Hyzop
T. Zulfa otu; Çördük otu

365. Iberis amara
E. Bitter Candytuft
F. Ibérite blanche; Thlapsi
blanc
G. Bittere Schleifenblume
S. Blomsteriberis
Sp. Carraspique
It. Iberide bianco; Raspo amaro
Gr. Ibíris
Gr. Ιμπίρις
H. Tatárvirág
P. Ubiorek gorski
T. Dügümotu; Hunkarçiçeği

366. Ilex aquifolium
E. Holly
F. Houx
G. Stechpalme
S. Järnek
Sp. Acebo; Brusco
It. Agrifoglio
Gr. Lióprino
Gr. Λιόπρινο
H. Magyal; Krisztustövis
P. Ilwa; Ostrokrzew
T. Dikenli defne; Çoban puskülü

367. Ilex paraguariensis
E. Maté
F. Maté; Houx maté
G. Mate
S. Mate
Sp. Yerba mate
It. Yerba Mate cruz de Malta
Gr. Maté
Gr. Ματέ

H. Paraguayi tea
P. Ostrokrzew paragwajski
T. Paragua çayı; Mate

368. Ilicium verum
E. Star Anise
F. Anis étoile
G. Sternanis
S. Stjärnanis
Sp. Anis estrellado
It. Anice stellata
Gr. Ghlykániso to asterómorfo;
　Asteroídhes
Gr. Γλυκάνισο το αστερόμορφο·
　Αστεροϊδές
H. Csillag-ánizs
P. Badian właściwy
T. Çin anasonu; Yıldız anasonu

369. Impatiens noli-tangere
E. Touch-me-not
F. Ne-me-touchez-pas; Impatient
G. Springkraut; Rührmichnichtan
S. Sprinkorn
Sp. Nometoques
It. Non-mi-tocare
Gr. Mi- mou- áptou; Impásien
Gr. Μη-μου-άπτου· Ιμπάσιεν
H. Nebáncsvirág
P. Niecierpek; Nietykałek
T. Camgüzeli; Yabani kina çiç.

370. Indigofera tinctoria
E. Indigo
F. Indigo
G. Indigo
S. Indigo
Sp. Indigo; Anil
It. Indaco

Gr. Indhikokýanos; Loulaki
Gr. Ινδικοκύανος· Λουλάκι
H. Indigókék
P. Indygowiec barwierski
T. Çivit fidanı; Çivit ağacı

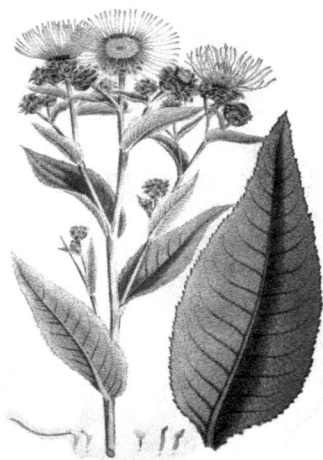

371. Inula helenium
E. Elecampane
F. Aunée
G. Alant
S. Alant; Ålandsrot
Sp. Enula
It. Enula
Gr. Inoula; Elénios
Gr. Ίνουλα; Ελένιος
H. Örvénygyökér; Perenizs
P. Oman wielki; Dziewiosił
T. İnduz otu; Andız otu

372. Ipomoea purpurea
E. Morning Glory
F. Étoile du matin; Ipomée
G. Kaiserwinde
S. Purpuvinda

Sp. Maravillas
It. Sciarapa
Gr. Ipoméa
Gr. Ιπομέα
H. Kerti folyondár
P. Wilec
T. Kahkaha çiç.; Gündüz sefası

373. *Iris florentina*
E. Iris; Orris Root
F. Iris de florence; Iris flambé
G. Schwertlilie
S. Trädgårdsiris
Sp. Lirio florentino
It. Giaggiolo; Iride; Ireos
    florentina
Gr. Iris i florentiáni; Krínos;
    Iridha
Gr. Ίρις η φλορεντιάνη˙ Κρίνος˙
    Ίριδα
 H. Irisz; Nőszirom
P. Kosaciec floreńtynski;
    Fiołkowy korzeń
T. Mavi zambak; Mavi Süsen

374. *Iris pseudacoros*
E. Yellow Flag
F. Iris faux-acore
G. Wasser-Schwertlilie
S. Svärdslilja
Sp. Acoro bastardo
It. Giglio d'acqua
Gr. Nerókrinos;
    Psevdhákoros
Gr. Νερόκρινος˙ Ψευδάκορος
H. Sárga nőszirom
P. Kosaciec żółty
T. Navruzu (bataklık)

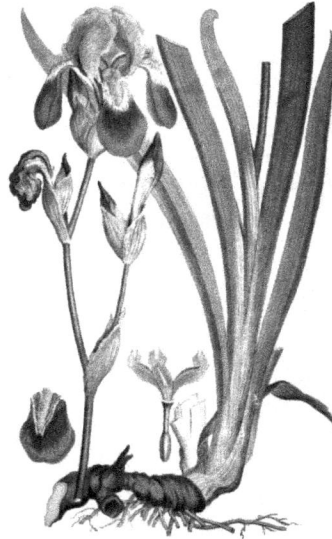

375. *Iris versicolor*
E. Blue Flag
F. Iris multicolor
G. Bunte Schwertlilie
S. Brokiris
Sp. Lirio multicolore
It. Giaggiolo multicolore
Gr. Iridha i pikilóchromi
Gr. Ίριδα η ποικιλόχρωμη
H. Foltos nőszirom
P. Kosaciec pstry
T. Mor süsen

376. *Isatis tinctoria*
E. Woad
F. Guède; Herbe de St Philippe
G. Waid; Faberwaid
S. Vejde
Sp. Glasto; Hierba pastel
It. Guado; Glasto
Gr. Isátis

Gr. Ισάτις
H. Európai indigo
P. Siniło; Urzet
T. Çivit otu

377. Jasiminum officinalis
E. Jasmine
F. Jasmin
G. Jasmin
S. Jasmin
Sp. Jasmin
It. Gelsomino
Gr. Yasemí
Gr. Γιασεμί
H. Jazmin
P. Jaśmin
T. Yasemin çiç.

378. Jateorhiza palmata
E. Calumba
F. Columbe
G. Colombowurzel
Sp. Colombo
It. Colombo; Columba
Gr. Aetheóriza
Gr. Αιθιόριζα
H. Kolombógyökér

379. Jatropha manihot→
Manihot utilissima

380. Jessenia bataua
E. Bataua Palm;
    Seje
F. Pataoua
G. Sejepalme
Sp. Seje; Milpesos
Gr. Yessénia
Gr. Γεσσένια

381. Juglans cinerea
E. Butternut
F. Noix de beurre
G. Butterwalnuss
S. Grå valnöt
Sp. Nogal ceniciento
It. Noce cenerino
Gr. Karidhiá i tefrí
Gr. Καρυδιά η τεφρή
H. Amrikai vajdió
P. Orzech olejny
T. Ceviz yağı ağ.

382. Juglans regia
E. Walnut
F. Noix
G. Walnuss
S. Valnöt
Sp. Nogal
It. Noce
Gr. Karídhi
Gr. Καρύδι
H. Dió
P. Orzech
T. Ceviz

383. Juniperus communis
E. Juniper
F. Genièvre
G. Wacholder
S. En
Sp. Jinepro; Enebro
It. Ginepro
Gr. Kédhros;
    Aghriokiparíssi
Gr. Κέδρος˙ Αγριοκυπαρίσσι
H. Boróka
P. Jałowiec
T. Ardıç

384. Justicia adhadota
E. Malabar Nut
F. Noix de Malabar
G. Malabarnuss
S. Malabarnöt
Sp. Arusa; Nuez de Malabar
It. Noce del Malabar; Noce delle
   Indie
Gr. Iuostíkia i adhatódhi; Kariá
   Malabár
Gr. Ιουστίκια η αδατόδη˙ Καρυά
   Μαλαμπάρ

385. Kaempferia galanga→
Alpinia officinarum

386. Kalmia latifolia
E. Mountain Laurel
F. Laurier des montagnes; Kalmie
G. Lorbeerrose; Berglorbeer
S. Bredbladig kalmia
It. Allora di montagna
Gr. Kálmia i ghlafkí
Gr. Κάλμια η γλαυκή
H. Kalmia; Széleslevelű
P. Wozięczelina
T. Kalmiya; Defnegülü

387. Knautia arvensis
E. Field Scabious
F. Knautie des champs
G. Acker-Scabiose; Acker
   Witwenblume
S. Åkervädd
Sp. Escabiosa
It. Vedovella campestre, Orecchio
   d'asino
Gr. Knautiá i arouraía
Gr. Κναούτια η αρουραία

H. Ördögszem
P. Świerzbnica polna
T. Tarak otu

388. Krameria triandra
E. Rhatany
F. Kramerie triandre; Ratanhia
   du Péru
G. Krameria; Rhataniawurzel
S. Ratanhiabuske
Sp. Ratania; Raiz de los dientes
It. Ratania
Gr. Ratánia
Gr. Ρατάνια
H. Ratanhiagyőkér
P. Partwin
T. Ratanya

389. Laburnum anagyroides
E. Laburnum; Golden Rain
F. Pluie d'or; Cytise
G. Goldregen
S. Sydgullregn
Sp. Lluva de oro
It. Laburno
Gr. Lavoúrnon; Psíkantho
Gr. Λαβούρνον; Ψίκανθο
H. Aranyeső
P. Szczodrzeniec; Złotakap
   pospolity
T. Yalan abanoz ağ

390. Lactuca sativa
E. Lettuce
F. Laitue
G. Lattich
S. Sallad
Sp. Lechuga
It. Lattuga

Gr. Maroúli
Gr. Μαρούλι
H. Saláta; fejes
P. Sałata
T. Marul

391. Lactuca serriola
E. Prickly Lettuce
F. Laitue scarole
G. Stachel-Lattich
S. Taggsallat
Sp. Lechuga brava; Serallon
It. Lattuga selvatica
Gr. Prionófilo
Gr. Πριονόφυλλο
H. Vadsaláta
P. Sałata kompasowa
T. Yağ marulu

392. Lactuca virosa
E. Wild Lettuce; Lettuce Opium
F. Laitue vireuse
G. Giftlattich
S. Giftsallat
Sp. Lechuga silvestre; Lechuga
   virosa
It. Lattuga velenosa
Gr. Aghrio maroúli; Toxikí
   maroúli
Gr. Άγριο μαρούλι· Τοξικί
   μαρούλι
H. Mérges saláta
P. Sałata jadowita
T. Zehirli marul

393. Laminaria saccharina
E. Kelp
F. Laminaire
G. Blattang
S. Sockertång

Sp. Laminaria; Algas marinas
It. Laminaria
Gr. Feofíki
Gr. Φαιοφύκη
H. Tengeri moszat; Hínár
P. Listownica cukrowa
T. Lamininarya

394. Lamium album
E. White Deadnettle
F. Lamier blanc; Ortie blanche
G. Weisse Taubnessel
S. Vitplister
Sp. Ortiga blanca; Ortiga muerta
It. Lamio; Ortica bianca
Gr. Lámio
Gr. Λάμιο
H. Fehér árva csalán
P. Jasnota biała
T. Beyaz ballibaba

395. Lapsana communis
E. Nipplewort
F. Lampsane; Herbe aux
   mamelles
G. Rainkohl
S. Harkål
Sp. Lampsano
It. Lampsano; Grespignolo
Gr. Sphalagóhorto
Gr. Σφαλαγγόχορτο
H. Bojtorjánsaláta
P. Łoczyga pospolita
T. Şebrek; Meme otu

396. Larix decidua
E. Larch
F. Alerce; Mélèze
G. Larche
S. Lärk

Sp. Alerce
It. Lance
Gr. Lárix; Ághrio péfko
Gr. Λάριξ; Άγριο πεύκο
H. Vörösfenyő
P. Modrzew
T. Kara çam

397. *Laurus nobilis*
E. Bay Laurel
F. Laurier noble; Laurier d'Apollon
G. Lorbeer
S. Lager
Sp. Laurel
It. Lauro nobile; Alloro
Gr. Dáphni
Gr. Δάφνη
H. Babér
P. Wawrzyn
T. Defne; Tefne

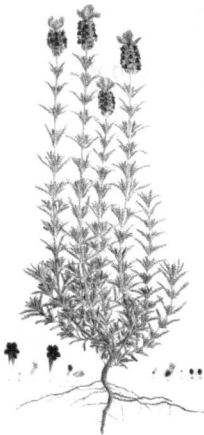

398. *Lavandula spp.*
E. Lavander
F. Lavande
G. Lavandel

S. Lavendel
Sp. Lavandula; Espliego
It. Lavanda
Gr. Levánda
Gr. Λεβάντα
H. Levendula
P. Lawenda
T. Lavanta çiç.

399. *Lavatera arborea*
E. Tree Mallow
F. Mauve des jardins; Lavatere
G. Malve
S. Jättemalva
Sp. Malva árbol
It. Malva
Gr. Dhendromolócha
Gr. Δενδρομολόχα
H. Papsajtfa
P. Ślazówka
T. Korkut

400. *Lawsonia alba/inermis*
E. Henna
F. Henne
G. Hennastrauch
S. Henna
Sp. Hena
It. Hennè rosso
Gr. Hénna
Gr. Χέννα
H. Henna
P. Henna
T. Kına ağ.; Hena ağ.

401. *Ledum palustre*
E. Labrador Tea; Marsh Ledum; Wild Rosemary
F. Romarin sauvage
G. Sumpf-Porst

S. Skvattram
Sp. Romero silvestre
It. Ledone
Gr. Lédhon eloharés
Gr. Λέδον ελοχαρές
H. Molyúző
P. Bagno; Rozmaryn czeski
T. Biberiye (yabani); Zehirli biberiye

402. Leonurus cardiaca
E. Motherwort
F. Agripaume
G. Herzgespann
S. Hjärtsilla
Sp. Agripalma
It. Cardiaca leonorus
Gr. Leonórous
Gr. Λεονόρους
H. Gyöngyatak; Oroszlánfark
P. Serdecznik
T. Aslan otu; Aslankuyruğu otu

403. Lepidium sativum
E. Garden Cress
F. Cresson alènois
G. Gartenkresse
S. Smörgåskrasse
Sp. Mastuerzo
It. Crescione; Agretto
Gr. Kárdhamo
Gr. Κάρδαμο
H. Kerti zsálya
P. Pieprzyca siewna; Rzeżucha siewna
T. Tere; Bahçeteresi

404. Levisticum officinalis
E. Lovage
F. Livèche; Ache des montagnes

G. Garten Liebstöckel
S. Libbsticka
Sp. Levistico; Apio de montaña
It. Sedano di montagna; Levistico
Gr. Levístiko
Gr. Λεβίστικο
H. Lestyán
P. Lubiśnik; Lubczyk
T. Selam otu; Kurtbağı; Şifalı selamotu

405. Ligusticum scoticum
E. Sea Lovage; Scots Lovage
F. Persil de mer; Angélique à feuilles d'ache
G. Meer Liebstöckel; Schottische Mutterwurz
S. Strandloka
Sp. Apio de mar
It. Ligustico di Scozia
Gr. Ligoustikó Skotías
Gr. Λιγουστικό Σκοτίας
H. Tengeri lestyán

406. Ligustrum vulgare
E. Privet
F. Troène vulgaire
G. Liguster
S. Liguster
Sp. Ligustro; Alheña
It. Ligustro
Gr. Ligoústron; Aghriomyrtyá
Gr. Λιγούστρον· Αγριομυρτιά
H. Fagyal
P. Ligustr pospolity
T. Kurtbağrı

407. Lilium candidum
E. White Lily; Madonna Lily
F. Lis; Lis de la Madone

G. Weisse Lilie; Madonnen Lilie
S. Madonnalilja
Sp. Azucena; Lirio de la Madona
It. Giglio
Gr. Leríon; Krínos
Gr. Λείριον· Κρίνος
H. Liliom
P. Lilia biała
T. Beyaz zambak

407α. Limonium carolinianum→Statice carolinianum

408. Linaria vulgaris
E. Toadflax
F. Linaire commune
G. Frauenflachs; Gemeines
   Leinkraut
S. Gulsporre
Sp. Pajarita; Linaria
It. Linaiolo; Urinaria
Gr. Linária
Gr. Λινάρεια
H. Gyújtoványfű
P. Lnica; Lnianka
T. Navruz otu; Yabani keten

409. Linum catharticum
E. Purging Flax
F. Lin Purgatif
G. Purgier-Lein
S. Vildlin
Sp. Lino catártico
It. Lino purgativo
Gr. Linó kathartikó
Gr. Λινό καθαρτικό
H. Törpe vadlen; Hashajtó
   tulajdonságú
P. Len przeczyszczający

T. Keten munki

410. Linum utitatissimum
E. Flax; Linseed
F. Lin cultivé
G. Flachs; Leinsamen
S. Lin
Sp. Lino; Linaza
It. Lino; Linosa
Gr. Línon; Linári
Gr. Λίνον· Λινάρι
H. Lenmag
P. Len
T. Keten

**411. Lippia citriodora→
Aloysia triphilla**

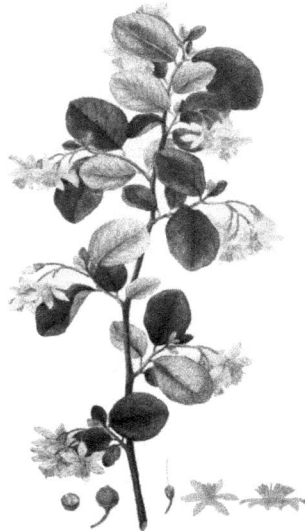

412. Liquid amber orientalis
E. Storax
F. Liquidambar; Styrax du
   Levant
G. Amberbaum

S. Storax
Sp. Liquidambar de oriente
It. Balsamo storace
Gr. Stýrax
Gr. Στύραξ
H. Stóraxfa; Stórax balszam
P. Ambrowiec; Oblewnik;
T. Günlük Ayıfındığı

413. *Liriodendron tulipifera*
E. Tulip Tree; Magnolia Tree
F. Tulipier de Virginie
G. Tulpenbaum
S. Tulpanträd
Sp. Tulipero de Virgina
It. Albero dei tulipani
Gr. Liriódhendhro
Gr. Λειριόδενδρο
H. Tulipánfa
P. Tulipanowiec
T. Amerika lale ağ

414. *Lithospermum officinalis*
E. Gromwell
F. Gremil; Herbe aux perles
G. Steinsame
S. Stenfrö
Sp. Litospermo
It. Migliarino; Litospermo
Gr. Lithóspermon; Dhadháki
Gr. Λιθόσπερμον· Δαδάκι
H. Kömag; Gyöngyköles
P. Nawrot
T. Taş kesen otu; İnci otu

415. *Lobaria pulmonaria*
E. Lungwort
F. Pulmonaire du chêne
G. Echte Lungenflechte

S. Lunglav
Sp. Pulmonaria de árbol
It. Polmonaria di quercia
Gr. Loboulária i poulmonária
Gr. Λομπουλάρια η
   πουλμονάρια
H. Tűdözuzmó
P. Granicznik
T. Akçiger likeni; Çigeryoğsunu

416. *Lobelia dortmanna*
E. Water Lobelia
F. Lobélie de Dortmann
G. Wasser-Lobelie
S. Notblomster
Sp. Lobelia acuatica
It. Lobelia acquatica
Gr. Nerolobélia
Gr. Νερολομπέλια
H. Vízi lobélia
P. Stroiczka jeziorna

417. *Lobelia inflata*
E. Lobelia; Indian Tobacco
F. Lobélie enflée; Tabac indien
G. Lobelien; Indianertabak
S. Läkelobelia
Sp. Lobelia; Tabaco indio
It. Lobelia inflata
Gr. Lobélia
Gr. Λομπέλια
H. Lobélia
P. Lobelia rozdęta
T. Lobelya

418. *Lolium temulentum*
E. Darnel; Ray Grass; Drake
F. Ivraie
G. Taumel-Lolch

S. Dårrepe
It. Zizzania; Lolio; Panevino
Gr. Lólio to methistikó
Gr. Λόλιο το μεθυστικό
H. Szédítő vadacs
P. Matonka; Matonóg; Życica roczna
T. Delice otu; Buğday delicesi

419. Lonicera caprifolium
E. Honeysuckle
F. Chèvrefeuille
G. Geissblatt
S. Kaprifol
Sp. Madre selva
It. Caprifoglio
Gr. Aghióklima; Aghiófilo
Gr. Αγιόκλιμα· Αγιόφυλλο
H. Lonc; Szulák
P. Wiciokrzew przewiercień; Kozi powój
T. Hanım eli

420. Lophophora williamsii
E. Peyote
F. Peyotl
G. Peyote
S. Giftkaktus
Sp. Peyote
It. Pejote, Echinocacto
Gr. Peyót
Gr. Πεγιότ
H. Texaszi kaktusz
P. Peyotl
T. Peyote

421. Lotus corniculatus
E. Bird's Foot Trefoil
F. Lotier corniculé

G. Gemeiner Hornklee
S. Käringtand
Sp. Cuernecillo
It. Ginestrino; Loto cornicolato
Gr. Lotós keratoïdhís; Drelokoúki
Gr. Λωτός κερατοειδής 'Ντρελοκούκκι
H. Szarvaskerep
P. Komonica
T. Serpik; Gazalboynuzu

422. Luffa cylindrica
E. Loofah
F. Louffa; Torchon; Éponge vegetale
G. Luffagurke; Schwammgurke
S. Luffa
Sp. Estropajo; Jaboncillo
It. Luffa
Gr. Loúffa
Gr. Λούφα
H. Luffaszivacs
P. Trukwa
T. Lif; Lif kabağı

423. Lupinus albus
E. White Lupin
F. Lupin blanc
G. Weisse Lupine
S. Vitlupin
Sp. Altramu
It. Lupino
Gr. Loúpino
Gr. Λούπινο
H. Fehér farkasbab
P. Łubin biała
T. Beyaz turmus; Termiye

424. *Lycopersicum esculentum*
E. Tomato
F. Tomate
G. Tomate
S. Tomat
Sp. Tomate
It. Pommodoro
Gr. Domáta
Gr. Ντομάτα
H. Paradicsom
P. Pomidor
T. Domates

425. *Lycopodium clavatum*
E. Clubmoss; Stag's Horn
F. Lycopode
G. Bärlapp; Keulen-Bärlapp
S. Mattlummer
Sp. Licopodio común
It. Licopodio; Stregonia
Gr. Lykopódhion
Gr. Λυκοπόδιον
H. Korpafű
P. Babimor; Widlak goździsty
T. Kurt ayağı; Kiprit otu

426. *Lycopus europaeus*
E. Bugleweed; Gypsywort; Water
   Horehound
F. Pied-de-loup;
   Chanvre d'eau
G. Wolfsfuss; Wolfstrapp
S. Strandklo
Sp. Menta de lobo
It. Marrubio acqatica
Gr. Lýkopos
Gr. Λύκοπος
H. Farkastalpfű
P. Karbieniec

T. Kurt otu; Kalkanbezı otu

427. *Lysimachia nemorum*
E. Yellow Pimpernel
F. Lysimaque de bois
G. Waldgelbiweiderich
S. Skogslysing
Sp. Muraje amarillo
It. Lisimachia di bosco
Gr. Anagalís kítrini
Gr. Αναγαλίς κίτρινη
H. Liszinká
P. Tojeść

428. *Lysimachia nummularia*
E. Moneywort; Creeping Jenny
F. Lysimaque nummulaire;
   Herbes aux écus
G. Munzkraut; Pfennigkraut
S. Penningblad
Sp. Hierba de la moneda
It. Erba soldina; Nummularia
Gr. Lysimáchion i ovolofóros
Gr. Λυσιμάχιον η οβολοφόρος
H. Pénzeslevelű liszinka;
   Inyújtófű
P. Tojeść rozesłana
T. Sarı kız out; Karga otu

429. *Lythrum salicaria*
E. Purple Loosestrife
F. Salicaire
G. Blutweiderich
S. Fackelblomster
Sp. Salicaria; Arroyuela común
It. Salicaria; Riparella
Gr. Salikária
Gr. Σαλικάρια
H. Füzény

P. Krwawnica
T. Hevhulma

430. Magnolia officinalis
E. Magnolia
F. Magnolia
G. Magnolie
S. Magnolia
Sp. Magnolia
It. Magnolia
Gr. Magnólia
Gr. Μαγκνόλια
H. Magnólia
P. Magnolia
T. Manolya

431. Mahonia aquifolium
E. Oregon Grape; Mountain
   Grape
F. Mahonia à feuilles de houx
G. Gemeine Mahonia
S. Mahonia
Sp. Mahonia
It. Berberi
Gr. Maónia
Gr. Μαώνια
H. Kerti mahonia
P. Mahonia
T. Mahonya

432. Malus communis
E. Apple
F. Pomme
G. Apfel
S. Apel
Sp. Manzana
It. Mela
Gr. Mílo
Gr. Μήλο
H. Alma

P. Jabłko; Jabłoń
T. Elma

433. Malus sylvestris
E. Crab-apple
F. Pomme sauvage
G. Holzapfel
S. Vildapel
Sp. Manzana silvestre
It. Mela selvatica
Gr. Aghriómilo
Gr. Αγριόμηλο
H. Vadalma
P. Jabłoń płonka
T. Yabani elma

**434. Malva neglecta/
Rotundifolia**
E. Dwarf Mallow
F. Mauve naine; Mauve négligée
G. Kleine Malve
S. Skär kattost
Sp. Malva común
It. Malva domestica
Gr. Molócha i atiméliti
Gr. Μολόχα η ατιμέλητη
H. Papsajtmályva
P. Ślaz zaniedbany
T. Kısa ebegümeci

435. Malva sylvestris
E. Common Mallow; Blue
   Mallow
F. Mauve sauvage
G. Wilde Malve
S. Rödmalva
Sp. Malva
It. Malva fiori blu
Gr. Molócha; Aghriomolócha
Gr. Μολόχα˙ Αγριομολόχα

H. Mályva
P. Ślaz dziki
T. Büyük ebegümeci

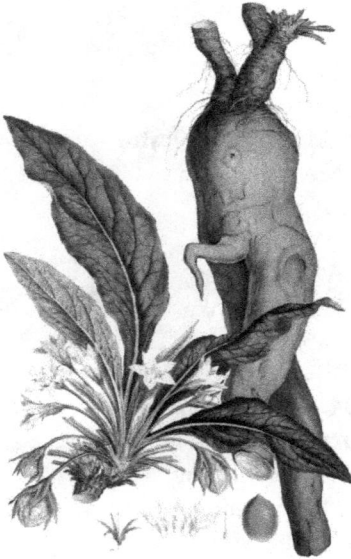

436. Mandragora officinalis
E. Mandrake
F. Mandragore
G. Alraun
S. Alruna
Sp. Mandrágora
It. Mandragora
Gr. Mandhragóras
Gr. Μανδραγόρας
H. Mandragora
P. Mandragora; Dziwostret
T. Hüngürük kökü; Adam kökü

437. Mangifera indica
E. Mango
E. Mangue
G. Mango

S. Mango
Sp. Mango
It. Mango
Gr. Mángo
Gr. Μάνγκο
H. Mangó
P. Mangowieć
T. Mangu; Hint kirazı

438. Manihot utilissima
E. Manioc; Tapioca; Cassava
F. Maniot douce; Kassave
G. Maniokstrauch
S. Maniok
Sp. Casaba; Tapioca
It. Manioca dolce
Gr. Kassáva; Tapióka
Gr. Κασσάβα· Ταπιόκα
H. Manióka
P. Kasawa; Manioc
T. Maniok; Tapioka

439. Maranta arundinacaea
E. Arrowroot
F. Maranta
G. Pfeilwurz
S. Arrowrot
Sp. Arraruz; Sagu
It. Fecola
Gr. Marántia; Arraroúti
Gr. Μαράντια; Αρραρούτι
H. Nyílgyökér
P. Arrowrot; Maranta
T. Ararot

440. Marrubium vulgare
E. White Horehound
F. Marrube blanc
G. Weisser Andorn

S. Kransborre
Sp. Marrubio blanco
It. Marrubio volgare
Gr. Marroúvio; Asproprasiá;
  Pikropáni
Gr. Μαρρούβιο˙ Ασπροπρασιά
  ˙Πικροπάνι
H. Orvosi pemetefű
P. Szanta pospolita
T. İt sineği; Bozotu; Köpek otu

441. Marsdenia condurango
E. Condurango
F. Condurango
G. Condurango
S. Kondurango
Sp. Condurango; Lechero
It. Condurango
Gr. Kondourángo
Gr. Κοντουράγκο
H. Kondurango cserje
P. Tojowiec condurango
T. Kondurango

**442. Matricaria
matricarioides→Chamomilla
suaveolens**

443. Matricaria recutita
E. German Chamomile
F. Vraie camomille; Petite
  camomile
G. Kamille; Echte Kamille
S. Kamomill
Sp. Manzanilla común
It. Camomilla
Gr. Hamomíli
Gr. Χαμομήλι
H. Kamilla

P. Rumianek
T. Alman papatyası;
  Babunek

444. Medicago sativa
E. Alfalfa; Lucerne
F. Alfalfa; Luzerne
G. Alfalfa; Luzerne
S. Alfalfa; Lusern
Sp. Alfalfa; Mielga
It. Erba medica; Alfa alfa
Gr. Alfalfa
Gr. Αλφάλφα
H. Lucerna
P. Lucerna
T. Kaba yonca

445. Melaleuca alternifolia
E. Tea Tree
F. Arbre à thé
G. Teebaum
S. Tea tree
Sp. Árbol de té
It. Albero del tè
Gr. Dendhro tsaiou
Gr. Δένδρο τσαγιού
H. Ausztrál teafa
P. Drzewo herbaciane
T. Çay ağacı

446. Melaleuca leucodendron
E. Cayeput
F. Cajeput
G. Kayeput
S. Kayeput
Sp. Cayeput
It. Cajeput
Gr. Kayapoút; Melaléfki
Gr. Καγιαπούτ˙ Μελαλέυκη

H. Kayeputfa
P. Kayaputa
T. Kayapüt

447. Melilotus officinalis

E. Melilot
F. Mélilot; Herbe aux mouches
G. Echter Steinklee
S. Gul sötväpling
Sp. Meliloto
It. Meliloto; Erba venturina
Gr. Melílotos
Gr. Μελίλοτος
H. Somkóró
P. Nostrzyk; Zwyczajny
T. Yonca; Kokulu yonca; Sarı yonca

448. Melissa officinalis

E. Lemon Balm; Balm
F. Mélisse; Citronelle
G. Melisse; Zitronenkraut
S. Citronmeliss; Hjärtsfröjd
Sp. Melisa
It. Melissa; Cedronella; Erba
    limone
Gr. Melissóhorto
Gr. Μελισσόχορτο
H. Mézfű; Orvosi citromfű
P. Melisa lekarska;
    Rojownik
T. Oğul otu; Melisa

449. Melittes melisophyllum

E. Bastard Balm
F. Mélisse des bois
G. Immenblatt
S. Honungsmynta
Sp. Toronjil silvestre
It. Melittide; Boca di lupe
Gr. Melítes

Gr. Μελίτης
H. Méhfű
P. Miodownik
T. Melez oğulotu; Pisoğulotu

450. Mentha aquatica

E. Water Mint
F. Menthe aquatique
G. Wasserminze; Bachminze
S. Vattenmynta
Sp. Menta inglesa; Menta acuatica
It. Menta acquatica
Gr. Ghlifonáki
Gr. Γλυφονάκι
H. Vízimenta
P. Mięta wodna
T. Su nanesi; Puzıne

451. Mentha piperata

E. Peppermint
F. Menthe poivrée
G. Pfefferminze
S. Pepparmynta
Sp. Menta piperita
It. Menta; Menta piperata
Gr. Menta
Gr. Μέντα
H. Borosmenta
P. Pieperzowa; Mięta
    pieperzowa
T. Biberi nane; İngliz nanesi

452. Mentha pulegium

E. Pennyroyal
F. Menthe pouliot
G. Polyminze; Frohkraut
S. Plejmynta
Sp. Poleo
It. Menta puleggio; Menta
    Romana

Gr. Fliskoúni
Gr. Φλησκoύνι
H. Csombormenta
P. Mięta polej
T. Yarpuz

453. Mentha spicata/viridis

E. Spearmint; Garden Mint
F. Menthe verte; Menthe de
   Notre Dame
G. Ährige-Minze; Grüne-Minze
S. Grönmynta
Sp. Hierbabuena; Menta verde
It. Menta dolce; Erba Santa Maria
Gr. Dhiósmos
Gr. Δυόσμος
H. Fodormenta
P. Mięta zielona
T. Nane

454. Menyanthes trifoliata

E. Bogbean; Buckbean; Marsh
   Trefoil
F. Tréfle d'eau; Ményanthe
G. Sumfklee; Fieberklee;
   Bitterklee
S. Vattenklöver
Sp. Trébol aquático
It. Trifoglio fibrino;
   Scarfano
Gr. Meníanthos
Gr. Μενίανθος
H. Vidrafű
P. Trojan; Bobrek trójlistkowy;
   Trzylistek
T. Su Yoncası

455. Mercurialis annua

E. Annual Mercury
F. Mercuriale annuelle

G. Einjähriges Bingelkraut
S. Grenbingel
Sp. Mercurial
It. Mercorella; Erba strega
Gr. Merkouriális
Gr. Μερκουριάλις
H. Merkfű; Egynyári szélfű
P. Szczyr roczny
T. Sultan otu; Yerfesleğeni

456. Mercurialis perinnis

E. Dog's Mercury
F. Mercuriale vivace
G. Ausdauerndes Bingelkraut
S. Skogsbingel
Sp. Mercurial perenne
It. Mercorella bastardo;
   Canina
Gr. Skilóhorto; Skaróhorto
Gr. Σκυλόχορτο · Σκαρόχορτο
H. Kutyatejfű
P. Szczyr trwały
T. Köpekmarulu

457. Mespilus germanica

E. Medlar
F. Nèfle
G. Mispel
S. Mispel
Sp. Nispola
It. Nespolo
Gr. Méspilo
Gr. Μέσπιλο
H. Naspolya; Lasponya
P. Niezpułka
T. Muşmula

458. Meum athamanticum

E. Spignel; Baldmoney
F. Méon; Fenouil des Alpes

G. Bärwurz
S. Björnrot
Sp. Meo; Hinojo ursino
It. Finocchiello
Gr. Méon
Gr. Μέον
H. Tömjénillat
P. Oleśnik
T. Ayı rezenesi

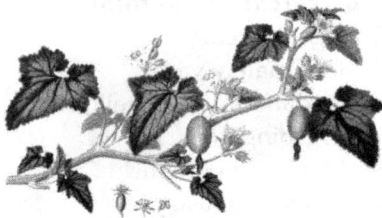

459. Momordica charantia
E. Balsam Pear; Bitter Gourd
F. Sorossie; Margou
G. Bittermelone
S. Bittergurka
Sp. Soubecoje
It. Cetriolo balsamina
Gr. Momordhíka i charántios
Gr. Μομορδίκα η χαράντειος
H. Sártök
P. Przepękla ogórkowata
T. Acayıp elması; Kudretnarı

460. Monardia didyma
E. Bergamot; Bee Balm;
    Oswego Tea
F. Bergamote; Monarde;
    Thé d'Oswego
G. Goldmelisse
S. Röd temynta
Sp. Bergamoto
It. Bergamotto

Gr. Monárdha
Gr. Μονάρδα
H. Bíbor ápolka
P. Pyznogłówka dwoista
T. Osveg çayı; Monard;
    Altınoğulotu

461. Monarda punctata
E. Horsemint
F. Monarde ponctuée
G. Monarda
S. Prickig temynta
Sp. Monarda
It. Monarda
Gr. Monárdha i stiktí
Gr. Μονάρδα η στικτή
H. Vadmenta; Lómenta
P. Mięta długolistna
T. Yabani nane

462. Morinda oleifera
E. Ben; Horseradish Tree
F. Moringa ailée
G. Pferderettichbaum
S. Pepparrotsträd
Sp. Maranga; Teberinto
It. Ghianda unguentaria;
    Noce di Behen
Gr. Moríndha i elaiofóros
Gr. Μορίνδα η ελαιοφόρος
H. Kék szantálfa
T. Ben; Surkun ağ.

463. Morus alba
E. White Mulberry
F. Mûre blanche
G. Weisse Maulbeere
S. Vittmullbär
Sp. Morera blanca
It. Mora di gelsa bianca

Gr. Aspromouriá
Gr. Ασπρομουριά
H. Fehér eper
P. Morwa biała
T. Beyaz dut

464. Morus nigra
E. Black Mulberry
F. Mûre noir
G. Schwarze Maulbeere
S. Svart mullbär
Sp. Morera negra
It. Mora di gelsa nero
Gr. Mavromouriá
Gr. Μαυρομουριά
H. Fekete eper
P. Morwa czarna
T. Kara dut

465. Musa spp.
E. Banana
F. Banane
G. Banane
S. Banan
Sp. Plátano
It. Banana
Gr. Banána
Gr. Μπανάνα
H. Banán
P. Banan
T. Moz

466. Musa sapientum
E. Plantain
F. Banane misquette
G. Kochbanane; Gemüsebanane
S. Kokbanan
Sp. Plátano; Plantanos machos
I. Banano
P. Figa rajska

467. Muscari comosum
E. Tassel Hyacinth
F. Muscari à grappes
G. Schopfige Traubenhyazinthe
S. Fjäderhyacint
Sp. Guitarilla; Jacinto penachuda
It. Muscari selvatico
Gr. Volvós
Gr. Βολβός
H. Fürtös gyöngyike
P. Szafirek miękkolistny
T. Arap sümbülü

468. Myrica cerifera
E. Bayberry; Wax Myrtle
F. Arbre à suif; Cirier;
    Myrica à cire
G. Wachsgagel; Wachsmyrte
S. Vaxpors
Sp. Mirica cerifera
It. Mirica
Gr. Psevdhomiríki kirofóros
Gr. Ψευδομυρίκη κηροφόρος
H. Viaszbokor
P. Woskorodny krzew
T. Mumağacı

469. Myristica fragrens
E. Nutmeg
F. Muscade
G. Muskatnuss
S. Muskotträd
Sp. Moscada
It. Noce moscata
Gr. Moschokáridho
Gr. Μοσχοκάρυδο
H. Szerecsendió
P. Gałka muszkatołowa
T. Küçük hindistan cevizi; Hint
    cevizi

470. *Myristica fragrans*
E. Mace
F. Macis
G. Muskatblütte
S. Muskotblomma
Sp. Macis
It. Macis
Gr. Floúdhi moschokáridhou;
　　Massís
Gr. Φλούδι μοσχοκάρυδου·
　　Μασσίς
H. Muskátvaj
P. Kwiat muszkatołowy
T. Muskat

471. *Myroxylon pereirae*
E. Peruvian Balsam
F. Baume de Perou
G. Peru Balsam
S. Perubalsamträd
Sp. Bálsamo del Peru
It. Balsamo del Peru
Gr. Myróxylo to Perouvianó
Gr. Μυρόξυλο το Περουβιανό
H. Perui balszam
P. Balsam peruwiański
T. Peru'nun balzam

472. *Myroxylon toluiferum*
E. Tolu Balsam
F. Baume de Tolu
G. Tolu Balsam
S. Tolubalsamträd
Sp. Bálsamo del Tolú
It. Balsamo del Tolu
Gr. Myróxylo to Tolouíforon
Gr. Μυρόξυλο το Τολουίφορον
H. Tolubalzsam
P. Balsam Tolu
T. Tolu'nun balzam

473. *Myrrhis odorata*
E. Sweet Cicely
F. Cerfeuil musqué
G. Süssdolde
S. Spansk körvel
Sp. Perifollo
It. Mirride
Gr. Seselis
Gr. Σεσελης
H. Spanyol turbolya
P. Marczewnik anyżowy;
　　Spąszyn
T. Misk maydonozu

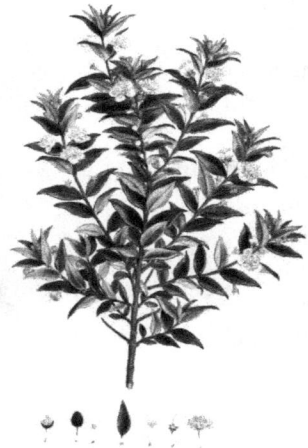

474. *Myrtus communis*
E. Myrtle
F. Myrte
G. Myrte
S. Myrten
Sp. Mirto; Arráyan
It. Mirto; Mortella
Gr. Mirtyá
Gr. Μυρτιά
H. Mirtusz
P. Mirt; Mirtyl

T. Mersin ağ

475. Nardostachys grandiflora
E. Spikenard
F. Nard Indien; Spiquenard
G. Nardenähre
S. Nardus
Sp. Nardo
It. Spignardi
Gr. Nardhostáchys
Gr. Ναρδοστάχυς
H. Nárdus
P. Spikanarda
T. Hint sünbulu

476. Nasturtium officinalis
E. Watercress
F. Cresson; Cresson de fontaine
G. Wassersenf; Brunnenkresse
S. Källfräne
Sp. Berro de agua
It. Crescione; Nasturzio
Gr. Nerokárdhamo; Kárdhamo
Gr. Νεροκάρδαμο· Κάρδαμο
H. Vízitorma
P. Rzeżucha wodna
T. Su teresi

477. Nelumba nocifera
E. Lotus
F. Lotus des Indes; Lotus sacré
G. Indischer Lotus
S. Indisk lotus
Sp. Loto sacrado
It. Loto d'Egitto
Gr. Lotós
Gr. Λωτός
H. Lotusz
P. Lotos
T. Hint lotusu; Lotus çiçeği

478. Nepeta cataria
E. Catmint
F. Herbe aux chats;
   Cataire
G. Katzen-Minze
S. Kattmynta
Sp. Nébeda; Hierba gatera
It. Erba dei gatti; Gattaia
Gr. Nepéta; Galeófilo
Gr. Νεπέτα· Γκαλεόφυλλο
H. Illatos macskamenta
P. Kocimięta
T. Nezle otu; Kedi nanesi otu

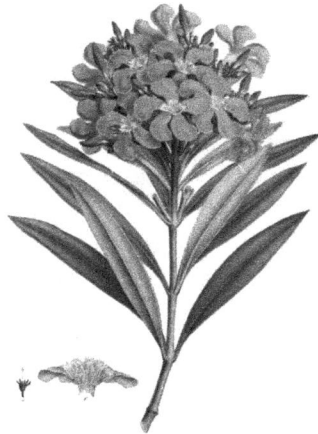

479. Nerium oleander
E. Oleander
F. Oléandre; Laurier-rose
G. Oleander
S. Oleander
Sp. Adelfa
It. Oleandro
Gr. Pikrodháfni
Gr. Πικροδάφνη
H. Oleánder
P. Oleander
T. Zekkum; Zıkkım

480. *Nicotiana tabacum*
E. Tobacco
F. Tabac
G. Tabak
S. Tobak
Sp. Tabaco
It. Tabacco
Gr. Kapnós
Gr. Καπνός
H. Dohány
P. Tytoń; Aprak
T. Tütün fıdanı

481. *Nigella sativa*
E. Love-in-a-mist; Black Cumin
F. Cumin noir; Nigelle
   aromatique
G. Schwarzer Kümmel
S. Svartkummin
Sp. Ajenuz; Comino negro
It. Nigella
Gr. Mávro kímino; Melánthion
Gr. Μαύρο κύμινο˙ Μελάνθιον
H. Fekete kömény
P. Czarnuszka siewna
T. Çörek otu; Karamuk sehniz

482. *Nymphaea alba*
E. White Water Lily
F. Nénuphar
G. Seerose; Seeblume
S. Vit näckros
Sp. Nenúfar blanco
It. Ninfea
Gr. Noúfaro
Gr. Νούφαρο
H. Fehér vizililiom
P. Wodna lilia; Grzybień białe
T. Nilüfer, Beyaz Nilüfer, Su Gülü

483. *Ocimum basilicum*
E. Basil
F. Basilic
G. Basilienkraut; Königskraut
S. Basilika
Sp. Albahaca; Alabega
It. Basilico
Gr. Vasilikós
Gr. Βασιλικός
H. Bazsalikom
P. Bazylia
T. Fesleğen; Rihan

484. *Oenanthe aquatica*
E. Water Dropwort
F. Oenanthe aquatique
G. Wasserfenchel
S. Vattenstäkra
Sp. Hinojo acuatico; Felandrio
   acuatico
It. Fellandrio
Gr. Oenánthi tou neroú
Gr. Οινάνθη του νερού
H. Borgyökér;
   Mételykóró
P. Kropidło wodne; Gałucha

485. *Oenothera biennis*
E. Evening Primrose
F. Onagre; Herbe-aux-ânes
G. Gemeine Nachtkerze
S. Nattljus
Sp. Onagra bienal
It. Onagra; Oenotera
Gr. Inóthira
Gr. Οινόθιρα
H. Ligetszépe; Csészekürt
P. Wiesiołek; Marzawa
T. Eşek çiç.

P. Wilżina ciernista
T. İdraotu; Kayıskıran

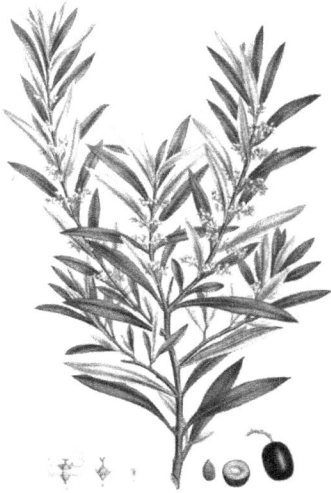

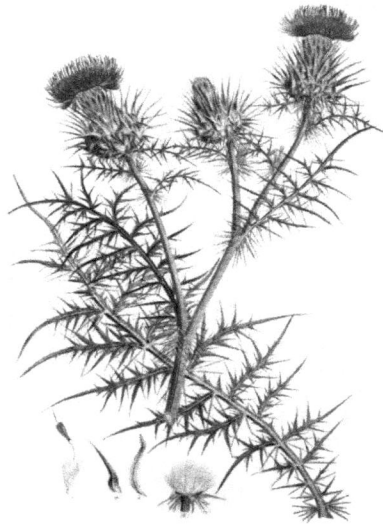

486. *Olea europaea*

E. Olive
F. Olive
G. Oliven
S. Oliv
Sp. Aceituna; Olivo
It. Oliva
Gr. Eliá
Gr. Ελιά
H. Olajfa
P. Oliwka
T. Zeytun; Zeytın

487. *Ononis spinosa*

E. Spiny Restharrow
F. Bugrane épineuse; Arrête-bœuf
G. Dornige Hauhechel
S. Bukstörne
Sp. Gatuña; Uñagata
It. Ononide spinosa; Stanca bue
Gr. Ononís
Gr. Ονωνίς
H. Iglice

488. *Onopordium acanthum*

E. Scotch Thistle; Cotton Thistle
F. Chardon écossais
G. Eselsdistel
S. Ulltistel
Sp. Alcachofa borriquero; Acanos;
    Cardo borriquero
It. Cardo di Scozia
Gr. Vodhinó agáthi
Gr. Βοδεινό αγκάθι
H. Szamárbogáncs
P. Popłoch; Oset podwórzowy
T. Galagan

489. *Opopanax chironium*

E. Opopanax
F. Opopanax; Panais sauvage
G. Gummi Pastinake; Wilde
    Pastinake

S. Söt myrra
Sp. Pánace
It. Oponaca; Panacea bastarda
Gr. Opopánax
Gr. Οπωπάναξ
H. Kentaurfű
P. Kosztywał
T. Kirkorazar; Opopanax

490. Opuntia ficus-indica
E. Prickly Pear; Indian Fig
F. Figue de Barbarie
G. Feigenkaktus
S. Fikonkaktus
Sp. Nopal; Chumero; Higo chombo
It. Fichi d'India
Gr. Fragosikiá
Gr. Φραγκοσυκιά
H. Fűgekaktusz
P. Figa indyjska
T. Hint inciri; Kaynana dili

491. Orchis mascula
E. Early Purple Orchid; Salep
F. Orchis-mâle
G. Manns-Knabenkraut; Stattliches Knabenkraut
S. Sankt Pers nycklar
Sp. Satirón manchado
It. Concordia
Gr. Orchidéa; Salépi
Gr. Ορχιδέα· Σαλέπι
H. Füles kosbor
P. Storczyk meski; Zieliulka
T. Hasieti sahleb

492. Origanum dictamos
E. Dittany of Crete
F. Dictame de Crète
G. Kretischer Diptam
S. Kretadiptam
Sp. Díctamo de Creta
It. Dittamo cretico
Gr. Dhíktamo
Gr. Δίκταμο
P. Trzemdata
T. Girit diktamı

493. Origanum majorana
E. Marjoram
F. Marjolaine
G. Majoran
S. Mejram
Sp. Mayorana; Mejorana
It. Maggiorana
Gr. Madzourána
Gr. Μαντζουράνα
H. Majoránna
P. Majeranek
T. Mercanköşk; Macuran çiçeği

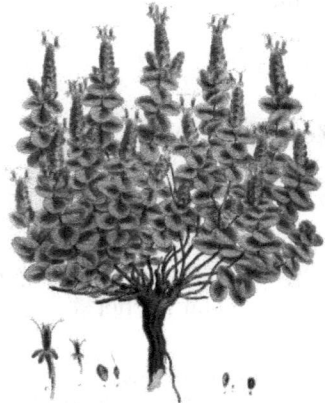

494. Oreganum vulgare
E. Oregano
F. Origan; Marjolaine sauvage

G. Oregano
S. Kungsmynta
Sp. Orégano
It. Oregano
Gr. Rígani
Gr. Ρίγανη
H. Szurokfű
P. Lebiodka
T. Keklik otu

495. Ornithogalum umbellatum
E. Star of Bethlehem
F. Dame d'onze heures
G. Doldiger Milchstern Stern von
   Bethlehem
S. Morgonstjärna
Sp. Leche de gallina
It. Bella di undiciore; Latte di
   gallina
Gr. Ornithogálo to skiadhanthés
Gr. Ορνιθόγαλον το
   σκιαδανθές
H. Ernyős madártej
P. Śniedek baldaszkowy
T. Şesiye çiçekli; Akyıldız sasal;
   Sunbala mariam

496. Oryza sativa
E. Rice
F. Riz
G. Reis
S. Ris
Sp. Arroz
It. Riso
Gr. Rízi
Gr. Ρύζι
H. Rizs
P. Ryż
T. Pirinc

497. Osmunda regalis
E. Royal Fern
F. Osmonde royale; Fougère
   royale
G. Königsfarn
S. Safsa
Sp. Afetos; Helecho real
It. Felce florida
Gr. Ftéri i vasilikí
Gr. Φτέρη η βασιλική
H. Király páfrány
P. Długosz królewski
T. Kral eğreltisi

498. Oxalis acetosella
E. Wood Sorrel
F. Pain-de-cocou; Petite oseille
G. Sauerklee
S. Harsyra
Sp. Acedera
It. Acetosella dei boschi
Gr. Xiníthra
Gr. Ξινίθρα
H. Madársóska
P. Szczawik zajęczy
T. Ekşi Yonca

499. Pœonia officinalis
E. Pæony
F. Pivoine officinale
G. Pfingstrose
S. Pion
Sp. Peonía; Hierba de
   Santa Rosa
It. Peonia
Gr. Peonía˙ Pighouniá
Gr. Παιωνία; Πηγουνιά
H. Peónia; Pünkösdi rózsa
P. Piwonia; Bujan

T. Ayı gülu; Şakayık

500. *Panax ginseng*
E. Ginseng
F. Ginseng
G. Ginseng
S. Ginseng
Sp. Ginseng
It. Ginseng
Gr. Tsinseng; Panax
Gr. Τσίνσενγκ; Πάναξ
H. Ginszeng
P. Żeńszeń
T. Ginseng

501. *Panicum miliaceum*
E. Millet
F. Millet
G. Hirse
S. Hirs
Sp. Mijo
It. Miglio; Panica
Gr. Kechrí
Gr. Κεχρί
H. Köles
P. Jagła; Proso zwyczajne
T. Dari

502. *Papaver rhoeas*
E. Field Poppy
F. Coquelicot; Pavot
G. Klatschmohn; Mohn
S. Kornvallmo
Sp. Amapola común
It. Papavero rosso
Gr. Paparoúna
Gr. Παπαρούνα
H. Mák; Pipacs
P. Mak; Maczek
T. Gelencik çiç; Yabanı haşhaş

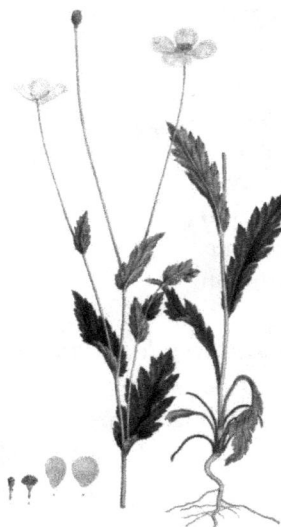

503. *Papaver somniferum*
E. Opium Poppy
F. Pavot somnifere; Opium
G. Schlafmohn
S. Opievallmo
Sp. Adormidera
It. Papavero d'oppio
Gr. Opio; Afióni
Gr. Όπιο˙ Αφιόνι
H. Ópium mák
P. Mak lekarski
T. Afyun çiç; Haşhaş

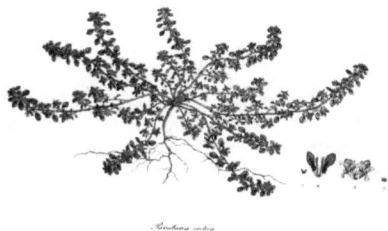

504. *Parietaria officinalis*
E. Pellitory-of-the-wall

F. Pariétaire; Épinard des
murailles
G. Glaskraut
S. Väggört
Sp. Parietaria ramiflora
It. Parietaria; Muraiola
Gr. Perdhikáki; Parietária
Gr. Περδικάκι· Παριετάρια
H. Falgyom
P. Pomurnik; Szlennicznik
T. Yapışkan otu; Sırça otu; Bere
otu

505. Paris quadrifolia
E. Herb Paris
F. Herbe de Paris; Raisin de
renard
G. Vierblättrige Einbeere;
Fuchstraube
S. Ormbär
Sp. Hierba de Paris; Uva de
Reposa
It. Erba crociona; Uva di volpe
Gr. Páris o tetráfilos
Gr. Πάρις ο τετράφυλλος
H. Farkasszőlő
P. Czworolist; Jedna jagoda
T. Tilki üzümü; Karga gőzű otu

506. Parnassia palustris
E. Parnassus Grass
F. Fleur du Parnasse; Foin du
Parnasse
G. Sumpfwiesenpflanze
S. Slåtterblomma
It. Gramigna di Parnasso
Sp. Parnasia
Gr. Parnássia i eloharís
Gr. Παρνάσεια η ελοχαρίς

H. Tőzegboglár
P. Dziewięciornik błotny
T. Parnasia çimi.

507. Passiflora incarnata
E. Passion Flower; Passiflora
F. Passiflore; Fleur de la passion
G. Passionsblume
S. Passionsblomma
Sp. Pasiflora; Maracuya; Flor de
pasion
It. Passiflora; Fiore della passione
Gr. Passiflóra
Gr. Πασιφλόρα
H. Golgotavirág
P. Męczennica
T. Çarkıfelek

508. Pastinaca sativa
E. Parsnip
F. Panais
G. Pastinak
S. Palsternacka
Sp. Chirivía
It. Pastinaca
Gr. Rápa; Révas
Gr. Ράπα· Ρέβας
H. Pasztinák
P. Pasternak
T. Yaban havucu

509. Paullinia cupana
E. Guarana
F. Guarana
G. Guarana
S. Guarana
Sp. Guaraná; Paulina;
Uaranziero
It. Guarana

Gr. Guarána
Gr. Γκουαράνα
H. Guarana-lián
P. Osmęta; Cierniopląt
T. Guarana

510. *Pedicularis palustris*
E. Lousewort
F. Herbe aux poux
G. Sumpf-Läusekraut
S. Kärrspira
Sp. Gallarito; Gorbiza
It. Pediculare
Gr. Psiróhorta; Pedhikouláris i eloharís
Gr. Ψειρόχορτο˙ Πεδικουλάρις η ελοχαρίς
H. Kakastaréj
P. Gnidosz
T. Çamur bitotu; Bit otu

511. *Pelargonium spp.*
E. Pelargonium
F. Pélargonium
G. Pelargonie
S. Pelargon
Sp. Geranio malva
It. Pelargonia
Gr. Pelarghónion
Gr. Πελαργόνιον
H. Muskátli
P. Pelargonia; Muszkatel
T. Itır çiç

512. *Persea americana*
E. Avocado
F. Avocat
G. Avocado

S. Avokado
Sp. Aguacate; Palta
It. Avocato
Gr. Avokádo
Gr. Αβοκάντο
H. Avokádo
P. Awokado
T. Avokado

513. *Petasites hybridus*
E. Butterbur
F. Chapeau du diable; Pétasite officinal
G. Pestwurz
S. Pestskråp
Sp. Petasites; Farfara; Sombrer
It. Erba dei tignosi; Petasites
Gr. Petasítis; Kolopána
Gr. Πετασίτης˙ Κωλοπάνα
H. Vörös acsalapu
P. Lepiężnik różowy
T. Veba kökü; Kafaotu

514. *Petroselinum crispus*
E. Parsley
F. Persil
G. Petersilie
S. Persilja
Sp. Perejil
It. Prezzemolo
Gr. Mydhanós
Gr. Μαϊδανός
H. Petrezelyem
P. Pietruszka
T. Maydanoz

515. *Peucedanum officinale*
E. Hog's Fennel; Sulphurwort
F. Persil des marais

G. Gebräuchlicher Haarstrang
S. Mästerrot
Sp. Ervatos; Rabo de
 puerco
 It. Finocchio di porco
Gr. Pefkedhánonto
 farmakeftikón; Ourá khiroú
Gr. Πεφσέδανον
 φαρμακευτικόν· Ουρά χοιρού
H. Disznókömény
P. Goryz błotny
T. Hınzır razıyanesi

516. *Peucedanum ostruthium*
E. Masterwort
F. Peucédane impératoire
G. Meisterwurz
S. Mästerrot
Sp. Imperatoria
It. Imperatoria vera
Gr. Ostránthio
Gr. Οστράνθιο
H. Mestergyökér;
 Mesterlapu
P. Gorysz miarz
T. Kıral otu

517. *Peumus boldo*
E. Boldo
F. Boldo
G. Boldo; Chilenischer
S. Boldo
Sp. Boldo
It. Boldo del Cile
Gr. Bóldo
Gr. Μπόλντο
H. Boldó levél
P. Boldo
T. Boldu

518. *Pfaffia paniculata*
E. Pfaffia; Sumo
F. Ginseng de l'amazone
G. Amazonischer
 Ginseng
S. Suma
Sp. Suma; Ginseng
 brazilero
It. Pfaffia
Gr. Pfáfia i fovoidhís
Gr. Πφάφια η φοβοειδής
H. Brazil ginszeng
P. Suma korzeń

519. *Phaseolus vulgaris*
E. Bean
F. Haricot
G. Bohne
S. Böna
Sp. Haba; Judía
It. Fagiolo
Gr. Fassóli
Gr. Φασόλι
H. Bab
P. Fasola
T. Fasulya

520. *Phoenix dactylifera*
E. Date
F. Datte
G. Datel
S. Dadel
Sp. Datil
It. Dattero
Gr. Hourmás
Gr. Χουρμάς
H. Datolya
P. Daktyl
T. Hurma

521. *Phyllitis scolopendrium*
E. Hart's Tongue Fern
F. Langue-de-cerf; Scolopendre
G. Hirschzunge
S. Hjorttunga
Sp. Lengua de ciervo
It. Lingua cervina
Gr. Scolopéndrio
Gr. Σκολοπένδριο
H. Közönséges gimpáfrány
P. Języcznik
T. Geyik dili

522. *Physalis alkagengi*
E. Chinese Lantern; Winter
    Cherry
Fr. Alkékenge; Coqueret;
    Lanterne
G. Judenkirsche
S. Judekörs
Sp. Alquequenje; Uchuva;
    Halicabalo
It. Alchechengi; Chichingero;
    Palloncini
Gr. Phýsalis; Kerasoúli
Gr. Φυσαλίς· Κερασούλι
H. Zsidócseresznye
P. Miechownica; Miechunka
T. Güvey feneri; Çin feneri

523. *Physostigma venosum*
E. Calabar Bean
F. Fève de Calabar
G. Kalabarbohne;
    Gottesurteilbohne
S. Kalabarböna
Sp. Haba de Calabar
It. Fava di Calabar
Gr. Kýamos tou Kalavár

Gr. Κύαμος του Καλαβάρ
H. Kalabar baklasi
P. Fasola kalabarska

524. *Phytolacca decandra*
E. Pokeroot
F. Phytolaque; Raisin
    d'Amerique
G. Kermesbeere
S. Kermesbär
Sp. Hierba carmín; Fitolaca;
    Calalu
It. Fitolacca; Uva d'America;
    Cremesina
Gr. Phytoláka; Aghrio stafidha
Gr. Φυτολάκα· Άγρια σταφίδα
H. Alkörmös
P. Alkiermes
T. Şereçi boyası otu

525. *Picea abies*
E. Spruce
F. Sapin; Épinette; Épicéa
G. Rot-Tanne
S. Gran
Sp. Picea
It. Pece
Gr. Eríthrelati; Pikéa
Gr. Ερυθρελάτη;
    Πικέα
H. Lucfenyő
P. Świerk pospolity
T. Avrupa ladini

526. *Picrasma excelsa*
E. Quassia; Bitter Ash
F. Quassia; Simaroube
G. Quassia Holzspäne
S. Bitterved

Sp. Cuasia; Simaruba
It. Quassia; Simaruba
Gr. Kouássia
Gr. Κουάσια
H. Kvassziafa
P. Kwasja

527. Pilocarpus jaborandi
E. Jaborandi
F. Jaborandi
G. Jaborandi
S. Jaborandi-buske
Sp. Jaborandi; Juarandi; Arruda
  brava
It. Giaborandi
Gr. Dzaborándi; Pilókarpos
Gr. Ντζαμποράντι·
  Πιλόκαρπος
H. Pilokarpus bokor levelei
P. Potoślin jaborandi

528. Pimenta officinalis
E. All-spice
F. Quatre-épices
G. Nelkenpfeffer
S. Kryddpeppar
Sp. Pimienta gorda; Pituca
It. Pepe garofanato; Pimento
Gr. Bahári
Gr. Μπαχάρι
H. Szegfűbors
P. Pimenta lekarska
T. Bac biber; Jamayıka biber;
  Yenibahar

529. Pimpinella anisum
E. Aniseed
F. Anis
G. Anis

S. Anis
Sp. Anis verde
It. Anice
Gr. Ghlikániso
Gr. Γλυκάνισο
H. Anizs
P. Anyź
T. Anason; Anasun

530. Pimpinella saxifraga
E. Burnet Saxifrage
F. Petit boucage; Boucage
  saxifrage
G. Kleine Bibernelle
S. Bockrot
Sp. Pimpinela
It. Sanguisorba; Pimpinella
Gr. Pimpinélla i saxifrágha
Gr. Πιμπινέλλα η σαξιφράγα
H. Rákfarkfű; Bábafű; Csabafű
P. Biedrzeniec mniejszy
T. Taş anasonu; Abdest bozan otu

531. Pinguicula vulgaris
E. Butterwort
F. Grassette vulgaire
G. Gemeines Fettkraut
S. Tätört
It. Pinguicola; Erba da taglio
Gr. Pingouíkoula
Gr. Πιγγουίκουλα;
H. Hízóka
P. Tłustosz
T. Semizotu

532. Pinus halapensis
E. Aleppo Pine
F. Pin d'Aleppe
G. Italienische Kiefer

S. Aleppotall
It. Pino Calabrese
Gr. Péfko
Gr. Πεύκο
H. Aleppói fenyő
T. Halep çam

533. *Pinus pinea*
E. Stone Pine; Umbrella Pine
F. Pin pignon
G. Italienische Steinkiefer
S. Pinje
Sp. Pino piñonero
It. Pino d'Italia
Gr. Koukounariá
Gr. Κουκουναριά
H. Pignoli fenyő; Mandula fenyő
P. Pinioły
T. Çam fıstık; Fıstığı ağacı

534. *Pinus silvestris*
E. Scotch Pine
F. Pin silvestre
G. Wald-Kiefer
S. Vanlig tall
Sp. Pino albar; Pino montaña
It. Pino silvestre
Gr. Péfko to kinó; Pinós
Gr. Πεύκο το κοινό˙ Πινός
H. Erdei fenyő
P. Sosna
T. Sarı çam

535. *Piper angustifolium*
E. Matico; Soldier's Herb
F. Matico; Arthante allongée
G. Soldatenkraut
S. Smalbladet peber/Soldaterurt
Sp. Matico; Cordoncillo

It. Matico; Erba di Soldato
Gr. Matíkon
Gr. Ματίκον
H. Keskenylevelű bors
T. Filfil; Matiko

536. *Piper betel*
E. Betel
F. Bétel
G. Betel
S. Betel
Sp. Betel
It. Betel
Gr. Bétel; Pipéri betelión
Gr. Βετέλ˙ Πιπέρι βετέλιον
H. Bétel bors
P. Betel indyjska; Pieprz żuwny
T. Tanbul; Betel; Hint asmasi

537. *Piper methysticum*
E. Kava-Kava; Intoxicating
   Pepper
F. Kawa-Kawa
G. Kavapfeffer
S. Kava
Sp. Kava
It. Kavakava
Gr. Káva pipéri
Gr. Κάβα πιπέρι
H. Kava
P. Kawa-Kawa
T. Kava biberi

538. *Piper nigrum*
E. Black Pepper
F. Poivre noir
G. Schwarzer Pfeffer
S. Peppar
Sp. Pimienta negra

It. Pepe nero
Gr. Mávro pipéri
Gr. Μαύρο πιπέρι
H. Fekete bors
P. Czarny pieprz
T. Siyah biber; Karabiber

539. *Piscadia erythrina/*
Piscipula
E. Piscidia; Fish Poison Bark;
Jamaican Dogwood
F. Bois-ivrant; Cornouiller
G. Fischrindenbaum;
Kornelbaum
S. Piscadia
Sp. Piscidia; Palo emborrachador;
Comiro
It. Corniola;
Piscadia
Gr. Piskádia i erythríni
Gr. Πισκάντια η
ερυθρίνη

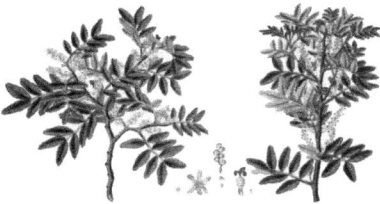

540. *Pistacia lentiscus*
E. Mastic
F. Mastic; Lentisque
G. Mastix
S. Mastixbuske
Sp. Lentisco; Masilla
It. Mastice Greco
Gr. Mastícha
Gr. Μαστίχα

H. Masztix; Ragasztómézga
P. Lentyszek; Mastyxowe
drzewo
T. Damla sakızı ağ.; Meneviş ağ.

541. *Pistacea vera*
E. Pistachio
F. Pistache
G. Pistazie
S. Pistaschmandel
Sp. Pistacho
It. Pistaccio
Gr. Fistíki
Gr. Φιστίκι
H. Pisztácia
P. Pistacja; Pistazie
T. Şam fıstık

542. *Pisum sativum*
E. Pea; green
F. Pois; vert
G. Erbse
S. Ärt
Sp. Guisante
It. Pisello
Gr. Arakás
Gr. Αρακάς
H. Borsó
P. Groch
T. Bezelye

543. *Plantago lanceolota*
E. Ribwort Plantain
F. Plantain lancéolé
G. Spitzer Wegerich
S. Svartkämper
Sp. Llantén menor
It. Piantaggine
Gr. Eptánevro

Gr. Επτάνευρο
H. Lándzsás útifű
P. Babka lancetowata; Skołojrza;
T. Dar yapraklı sinirli otu

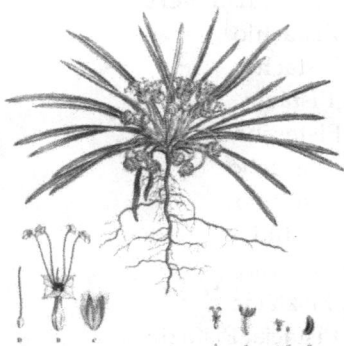

544. *Plantago major*
E. Greater Plantain
F. Plantain majeur; Grand
plantain
G. Grosser Wegerich;
Breitblätriger Wegerich
S. Groblad
Sp. Llantén mayor; Lengua de
carnero
It. Piantaggine grande
Gr. Pendánevro
Gr. Πεντάνευρο
H. Nagy útifű
P. Babka zwiczajna
T. Sinir otu

545. *Plantago ovata*
E. Iphagula
F. Isphagula
G. Spogel Wegerich
S. Vitt loppfrö
Sp. Isfágula; Ispágula

It. Isfagula
Gr. Isfagoúla
Gr. Ισφαγκούλα
H. Iszfagúla
P. Babka jajowata
T. İspağul otu

546. *Plantago psillium*
E. Psyllium
F. Plantain pulicaire
G. Flohsamen; Heusamen
S. Loppfrö
Sp. Zaragatona
It. Psillio
Gr. Psyllóhorto; Vedouróhorta
Gr. Ψιλλόχορτο Βεντουρόχορτο
H. Bolhamag
P. Babka płesznik
T. Karnıyarık

547. *Platanos hispanica/ Orientalis*
E. London Plane; Oriental Plane
F. Platane
G. Platane
S. Orientalisk platan
Sp. Plátano
It. Platano
Gr. Plátanos
Gr. Πλάτανος
H. Platán
P. Platan
T. Çınar ağ; Ğavlağan ağ

548. *Plumbago europaea*
E. Leadwort
F. Dentelaire d'Europe
G. Bleiwurz
S. Blyblomma

Sp. Belesa
It. Piombaggine
Gr. Lepidhóhorton
Gr. Λεπιδόχορτον
H. Kékgyökér
P. Ołtewnik; Ołwianka
T. Diş otu; Karakına

549. Podophyllum peltatum
E. American Mandrake
F. Podophylle pelté
G. Entenfuss; Maiapfel
Sp. Mandraque americano;
   Podófilo
It. Podofillo
H. Amerikai tojásbogyó
P. Biedrzga tarczowata

550. Pogestemon patchouli
E. Patchouli
F. Patchouli
G. Patchouli
S. Patchouli
Sp. Pacholi; Cablan
It. Pacciuli
Gr. Patsoulí
Gr. Πατσουλί
H. Pacsulicserje
P. Paczułka
T. Silhat; Paçouli

551. Polemonium reptans
E. Abcess Root; Greek Valerian
F. Polémonie; Valerian
   Grecque
G. Griechischer Baldrian;
   Himmelsleiter
S. Krypblågull
Sp. Valeriana Griega

It. Valeriana greca; Polemonio
   striciante
Gr. Polemónio to érpon
Gr. Πολυμώνιο το έρπον
H. Kúszó csatvirág
P. Wielosił; Poziołek
T. Yunan kedi otu

552. Polygala amara
E. Dwarf Milkwort
F. Polygala amér
G. Bittere Kreuzblume
S. Bittert jungfrulin
Sp. Poligala amargor
It. Poligala amara
Gr. Polýgalon pikró
Gr. Πολύγαλον πικρό
H. Keserű pacsirtafű
P. Krzyżownica gorska

553. Polygala senega
E. Snakeroot; Senega
F. Sénéga; Laitier; Polygala
G. Senega
S. Senegarot
Sp. Senega; Serpentaria Senegales
It. Poligala senega
Gr. Polýgalon to Virghinión
Gr. Πολύγαλον το Βιργίνιον
H. Szenegafű
P. Krzyżownica wirginijska
T. Vergina süt otu; Senega

554. Polygala vulgaris
E. Common Milkwort
F. Polygala commun
G. Kreuzblume
S. Jungfrulin
Sp. Poligala

It. Poligala nostrale; Bozzolino
Gr. Polýgalon to kinón
Gr. Πολύγαλον το κοινόν
H. Hegyi pacsirtafű
P. Krzyżownica błotny
T. Süt otu

555. Polygonatum odoratum
E. Solomon's Seal
F. Sceau de Salomon
G. Gemeine Weisswurz;
    Salomonssiegal
S. Getrams
Sp. Sello Salomón; Poligonato
It. Sigillo di Salomone
Gr. Polyghonáto; Sfragídha tou
    Solomóndos
Gr. Πολυγονάτο· Σφραγίδα του
    Σολομώντος
H. Salamon pecsétje
P. Kokoryczka wonna
T. Mühür Suleyman Buğunluca
    otu

556. Polygonum aviculare
E. Knotgrass
F. Centonode; Renouée des
    oiseaux
G. Vogelknöterich
S. Trampört
Sp. Centinodia
It. Centinodia; Corregiola
Gr. Polýkombo
Gr. Πολύκομπο
H. Madárkeresfű; Disznópázsit
P. Rdest ptasi
T. Köyotu; Kadımalak

557. Polygonum bistorta
E. Bistort

F. Renouée bistorte
G. Natterknöterich; Natterwurz
S. Stor omrot
Sp. Bistorta; Hierba sanguinaria
It. Bistorta
Gr. Polýkombo bistórta
Gr. Πολύκομπο μπιστόρτα
H. Kígyógyökerű keserűfű
P. Rdest wężownik
T. Kurt pençesı; Çıyançik; Çimen
    eveleği

558. Polygonum hydropiper
E. Water Pepper; Smartweed
F. Curage; Poivre d'eau
G. Pfeffer knöterich
S. Bitterpilört
Sp. Pimienta acuática
It. Poligono
Gr. Idhropépero
Gr. Υδροπέπερο
H. Vízibors
P. Wodny pieprz; Rdest
    ostrogorzki
T. Su biberi

559. Polygonum persicaria
E. Redleg; Redshank; Common
    Persicaria
F. Pied rouge; Renouée
    persicaire
G. Pfirsichblättriger Knöterich
S. Pilört
Sp. Persicaria; Duraznillo
It. Salcerella
Gr. Agriopiperiá
Gr. Αγριοπιπεριά
H. Baracklevelű keresfű
P. Rdest plamisty
T. Söğüotu

560. *Polypodium vulgare*
E. Adder's Fern; Brake Root
F. Polypode commun
G. Tüpfelfarn; Engelsüss
S. Stensöta
Sp. Polipodio; Filipodio;
    Calaguala
It. Felce dolce; Polipodio
Gr. Polypódhi; Dhendhroftéri
Gr. Πολυπόδι˙ Δενδροφτέρη
H. Édesgyökerű páfrány
P. Paproć
T. Eğrelti otu

561. *Populus alba*
E. White Poplar
F. Peuplier blanc
G. Silber Pappel
S. Silverpoppel
Sp. Álamo blanco
It. Pioppo bianco
Gr. Léfki
Gr. Λεύκη
H. Fehér nyár
P. Topola biała
T. Ak kavak; Ak toz

562. *Populus candicans*
E. Poplar Buds; Balm of Gilead
    Buds; Tacamohaca
F. Peuplier del'Ontario
G. Weissliche Pappel; Grau
    Pappel
S. Ontariopoppel
Sp. Chopo de Canada
It. Pioppo del Ontario
Gr. Léfki i ipólefki
Gr. Λεύκη η υπόλευκη
H. Ontario nyárfa
P. Topola balsamiczna

563. *Populus nigra*
E. Black Poplar
F. Peuplier noir
G. Schwarz Pappel
S. Svart poppel
Sp. Álamo negro
It. Pioppo nero
Gr. Kaváki
Gr. Καβάκι
H. Fekete nyár
P. Topola czarna
T. Kara kavak; Kara toz

564. *Populus tremula*
E. Aspen
F. Peuplier tremble
G. Espe; Zitterpappel
S. Asp
Sp. Álamo temblón
It. Pioppo tremolo
Gr. Léfki i trémousa
Gr. Λεύκη η τρέμουσα
H. Rezgőnyár
P. Osa; Osika
T. Titrik kavak

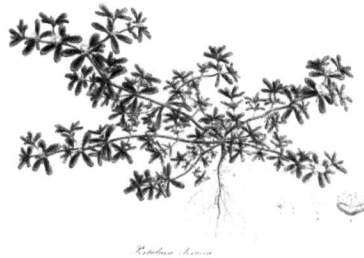

Portulaca oleracea

565. *Portulaca oleracea*
E. Purslane
F. Pourpier
G. Portulak; Burzelkraut
S. Portlak

Sp. Verdolaga
It. Porcellana
Gr. Andhrákla; Ghlistrídha
Gr. Ανδράκλα· Γλιστρίδα
H. Porcsin
P. Portulaka; Kurza noga
T. Pirpirim

566. *Potentilla anserina*

E. Silverweed
F. Potentille des oies;
   Ansérine
G. Gänsefingerkraut
S. Gåsört
Sp. Argentina; Plateada
It. Anserina
Gr. Potentílla
Gr. Ποτεντίλα
H. Liba pimpó
P. Pięciornik gęsi; Złotnik
T. Kaz gagası; Gümüş otu

567. *Potentilla erecta*

E. Tormentil
F. Tormentille
G. Ruhrwurz; Blutwurz
S. Blodrot
Sp. Tormentilla
It. Tormentilla
Gr. Tormentíla
Gr. Τορμεντίλα
H. Pimpófű
P. Pięciornik kurze ziele
T. Beşparmak otu; Kankökü

568. *Potentilla reptans*

E. Cinquefoil
F. Cinquefeuilles commun
G. Kriechendes Fingerkraut

S. Revfingerört
Sp. Cincoenrama; Quinquefolio;
   Cincoenflama
It. Cinquefoglie
Gr. Pendafiló
Gr. Πεντάφυλλο
H. Pimpó
P. Pięciornik rozłogowy
T. Reşatın otu

569. *Poterium sanguisorba*

E. Salad Burnet
F. Petite pimprenelle
G. Kleiner-Wiesenkopf
S. Äkta pimpinell
Sp. Hierba de cuchillo
It. Salvastrella
Gr. Potírio
Gr. Ποτίριο
H. Földi tömjén
P. Sowia strzała
T. Kücük mesine

570. *Primula elatior*

E. Oxslip
F. Primevère élevée
G. Hohe Primel; Schlüsselblume
S. Lundviva
Sp. Primula; Vellorita
It. Primula maggiore
Gr. Iranthés
Gr. Ιρανθές
H. Sugár kankalin
P. Pierwiosnka wyniosła
T. Çuhaçiçeği (buyuk)

571. *Primula Veris*

E. Cowslip; Paigle
F. Coucou; Primevère officinale

G. Echte Schlüsselblume
S. Gullviva
Sp. Gordolobollo; Flor de
primaver
It. Primula odorata
Gr. Prímoula i eariní; Paschalítsa
Gr. Πρίμουλα η εαρινή·
Πασχαλίτσα
H. Tavszi kankalin
P. Pierwiosnka lekarska;
Kluczyki
T. Tutya

572. Primula vulgaris
E. Primrose
F. Primevère vulgaire
G. Primel; Kissenprimel
S. Jordviva
Sp. Primavera
It. Primavera; Primula
Gr. Prímoula; Panayítsa;
Dhrakáki;
Gr. Πρίμουλα· Παναγίτσα·
Δρακάκι
H. Kankalin
P. Pierwiosnka bezłodygowa
T. Çuha çiçegi

573. Prunella vulgaris
E. Self Heal; All Heal
F. Brunelle commune
G. Kleine Braunelle
S. Brunört
Sp. Brunela; Consuelda menor
It. Brunella
Gr. Prounélla i kiní
Gr. Προυνέλλα η κοινή
H. Gyékfű; Gyikfű
P. Głowienka

T. Yara otu

574. Prunus armeniaca
E. Apricot
F. Abricot
G. Aprikose
S. Aprokos
Sp. Albaricoque
It. Albicocca
Gr. Veríkoko
Gr. Βερύκοκκο
H. Sárgabarack
P. Morela
T. Kayısı; Zerdali

575. Prunus avium
E. Gean; Wild Cherry
F. Mérisier des bois; Cerise
sauvage
G. Vogelkirsche; Süsskirsche
S. Sötkörsbär
Sp. Cereza silvestre; Albaruco
It. Ciliegio selvatico
Gr. Aghriokéraso
Gr. Αγριοκέρασο
H. Vadcseresznye
P. Czereśnia; Ptasia wiśnia
T. Yabani kiraz

576. Prunus cerasus
E. Sour Cherry; Morello Cherry
F. Griottier; Cerise aigre
G. Sauerkirsche
S. Surkörsbär
Sp. Guindal; Guindo garrafal
It. Amarena; Visciolo
Gr. Vísino
Gr. Βύσσινο
H. Meggy

P. Wiśnia
T. Vişne

577. Prunus domestica
E. Plum
F. Prune
G. Flaume
S. Plommon
Sp. Ciruela
It. Susina
Gr. Dhámaskino
Gr. Δαμάσκηνο
H. Szilva
P. Węgierka; Śliwa domowa
T. Erik

578. Prunus dulcis→
Amygdala dulcis
T.Kara keraz

579. Prunus laurocerasus
E. Cherry Laurel
F. Laurelle; Laurier-cerise
G. Kirschlorbeer
S. Lagerhägg
Sp. Cereza laurel
It. Lauro ceraso
Gr. Dhafnokerasiá
Gr. Δαφνοκερασιά
H. Babérmeggy
P. Laurowiśnia
T. Taflan ağ; Kara yemiş ağ

580. Prunus persica
E. Peach
F. Pêche
G. Pfirsch
S. Persika

Sp. Durazno; Melocotón
It. Pesca
Gr. Rodhákino
Gr. Ροδάκινο
H. Őszibarack
P. Brzoskwinia
T. Şeftali

581. Prunus serotina
E. Wild Cherry; Black Cherry
F. Cerise noire; Tardif
G. Schwarze Kirschen
S. Glanshägg
Sp. Cereza
It. Cigliegio tardivo
Gr. Mavrokéraso
Gr. Μαυροκέρασο
H. Cseresznye
P. Czeremcha amerykańska
T. Kara keraz

582. Prunus spinosa
E. Sloe; Blackthorn
F. Épine noir; Prunellier
G. Schlehe; Schwarzdorn
S. Slån
Sp. Endrina
It. Prugnolo
Gr. Tsapourniá;
    Aghriokorómilo
Gr. Τσαπουρνιά·
    Αγριοκορόμηλο
H. Kökény
P. Tarń
T. Dağ ereği; Çakal eriği

583. Psidium guayava
E. Guava

F. Pomme goyave
G. Guave
S. Guava
Sp. Guayabo
It. Guaia
Gr. Gouáva
Gr. Γκουάβα
H. Guajava
P. Gujawa
T. Hint armudu; Guava

584. Pulicaria dysenterica

E. Fleabane
F. Pulicaire dysentérique; Herbe
   Saint-Roche
G. Grosses Flohkraut; Ruhr
   Flohkraut
S. Loppörter
Sp. Pulicaria; Hierba de gato
It. Menta selvatica; Pulicaria
Gr. Poulikária
Gr. Πουλικάρια
H. Bolhafű
P. Płesznik
T. Pire otu

585. Pulmonaria officinalis

E. Lungwort
F. Pulmonaire officinale
G. Lungenkraut
S. Flacklungört
Sp. Pulmonaria
It. Polmonaria
Gr. Poulmonária
Gr. Πουλμονάρια
H. Orvosi tütőfű; Pettyegetett
P. Miodunka lekarska
T. Ciğer otu

586. Pulsatilla vulgaris→
Anemone pulsatilla

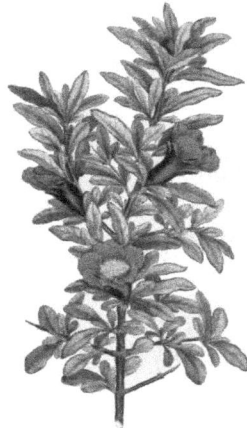

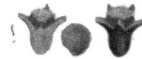

587. Punica granatum

E. Pomegranate
F. Grenade
G. Granatapfel
S. Granatäpple
Sp. Granado
It. Melagrano
Gr. Ródhi
Gr. Ρόδι
H. Gránátalma
P. Granat
T. Nar

588. Pyrola rotundifolia

E. Round-leaved Wintergreen
F. Pirole à feuilles rondes;
   Thé Suisse
G. Rundblättriges Wintergrün

S. Vitpyrola
Sp. Pírola
It. Piroletta a foglie rotonde
Gr. Pyróla i strogilófilli
Gr. Πυρόλα η στρογγυλόφυλλι
H. Egyvirágu körtike
P. Gruszyczka
  okrągłolistna
T. Emrud otu

589. *Pyrus communis*
E. Pear
F. Poire
G. Birne
S. Päron
Sp. Pera
It. Pera
Gr. Achládhi
Gr. Αχλάδι
H. Körte
P. Grusza
T. Armud

590. *Quassia amara*
E. Surinam Quassia;
  Bitterwood
F. Quassie amer; Bois
  de Surinam
G. Quassia; bitter
S. Surinam
  kvassia
Sp. Cuasia
It. Quassio
Gr. Kouássia pikró
Gr. Κουάσια πικρό
H. Keserűfa
P. Gorzkla
T. Acı ağac; Kuasia

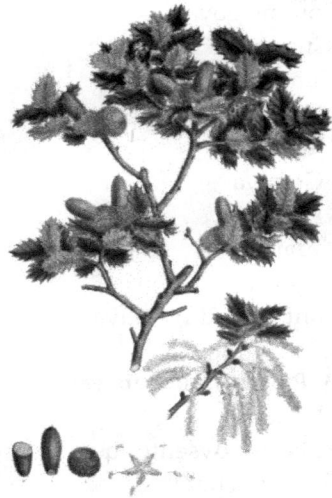

591. *Quercus macrolepsis*
E. Valonia Oak
F. Chêne vélani; Vélani
G. Wallonen Eiche
S. Valonia eken
It. Quercia vallonea
Gr. Pournári
Gr. Πουρνάρι
H. Kecskeszemű tölgy
P. Dąb Waloniji
T. Valona meşe ağ

592. *Quercus robur*
E. Common Oak
F. Rouvre; Chêne pédonculé
G. Stiel Eiche; Sommer Eiche
S. Ek
Sp. Roble
It. Quercia; Rovere; Quercia
  pelosa
Gr. Velanidhiá; Dhrís
Gr. Βελανιδιά· Δρύς

H. Tölgy
P. Dąb
T. Pelud meşesi; Kaya meşesi

593. *Quercus lusitanica*
Orientalis infectoria
E. Oak Gall
F. Chêne à galles
G. Gall Wespen
S. Aleppoek, Gallek, Galläppelek,
Sp. Agalla de roble
It. Noce galla
Gr. Dhriokikís; Kikís dhriós
Gr. Δρυοκηκίς· Κηκίς δρυός
H. Gubacs
P. Dąb żółć
T. Mazı Meşesi

594. *Ranunculus acris*
E. Buttercup
F. Bouton d'or; Jaunet
G. Butterblume; Scharfer
   Hahnenfuss
S. Smörblomma
Sp. Botón de oro; Ranuncolo
It. Ranuncolo
Gr. Ranoúnkoulos;
   Nerangoúla
Gr. Ρανούνκουλος·
   Νεραγκούλα
H. Boglárka
P. Jaskier ostry; Guzik złoty
T. Dügün çiç.; Turna ayağı;
   Kurbağa otu

595. *Ranunculus ficaria*
E. Pilewort; Lesser
   Celendine
F. Renoncule ficaire
G. Feigenwurzel

S. Svalört
Sp. Celidonia menor
It. Ficaria; Favagello
Gr. Zochadhóhorto;
   Spordharkéla
Gr. Ζωχαδόχορτο·
   Σπορδαρκέλα
H. Salátaboglárka
P. Ziarnopłon wiosenny
T. Basur otu

596. *Raphanus raphanistrum*
E. Wild Radish; Runch
F. Radis ravenelle
G. Acker Rettich
S. Åkerrättika
Sp. Rábano silvestre
It. Ravanello selvatico
Gr. Aghriorápano
Gr. Αγριοράπανο
H. Vad retek
P. Łpucha
T. Yabani turp

597. *Raphanus sativa*
E. Garden Radish
F. Radis cultivé
G. Rettich; Radieschen
S. Rättika
Sp. Rábano
It. Ravanello; Rafano nero
Gr. Rapanáki
Gr. Ραπανάκι
H. Retek
P. Murzynka; Rzodkiew
T. Turp; Ufak turp

598. *Rauwolfia serpentina*
E. Rauwolfia; Serpentwood
F. Rauwolfia; Arbre aux serpents

G. Rauwolfia
S. Rauvolfia
Sp. Rauvolvia; Aleli; Boboro;
   Guataco
It. Reserpina; Rauwolfia
Gr. Rauvólfia; Serpentína
Gr. Ραουβόλφια; Σερπεντίνα
H. Kígyós Vérnyomáscserje
P. Rauwolfia żmijowa; Zgrzyn
T. Yilan kökü; Rauvolfıya;
   Yilancalis

599. Rhamnus cathartica
E. Purging Buckthorn
F. Nerprun purgatif
G. Purgier-Kreuzdorn
S. Getapel
Sp. Espino cerval
It. Spinocervino
Gr. Rámnos i kathartikí
Gr. Ράμνος η καθαρτική
H. Varjútövis
P. Szakłak pospolity
T. Akdiken (yabani);
   Adi cehri

600. Rhamnus purshiana
E. Cascara
F. Écorce sacrée
G. Casteralrinde
S. Sagradabuske
Sp. Cáscara sagrada
It. Cascara sagrada
Gr. Kaskára sagrádha
Gr. Κασκάρα σαγκράδα
H. Kaszkarabokor
P. Szakłak amerykański;
   Kaskara
T. Akdiken (Amarika); Kaskara;
   Sagrada

601. Rheum officinalis
E. Medicinal Rhubarb
F. Rhubarbe officinale
G. Rhabarbar, Chinesischer
S. Läkerabarbar
Sp. Ruibarbo chino
It. Rabarbaro cina; Rabarbaro
   medicinale
Gr. Ríon to farmakeftikón
Gr. Ρήον το φαρμακευτικόν
H. Orvosi rebarbara
P. Rabarbar
T. Ravendi

602. Rheum rhaponticum
E. Garden Rhubarb
F. Rhubarbe; Rhubarbe anglaise
G. Rhapontikrhabarber
S. Munkrabarbar
Sp. Ruibarbo
It. Rabarbaro
Gr. Ríon; Ravénti
Gr. Ρήον· Ραβέντι
H. Rebarbara
P. Rabarbar ogrodowy
T. İngliz ravendi

603. Rhus glabra
E. Sweet Sumach; Smooth
   Sumach
F. Sumac
G. Sumach; Scharlach Sumach
S. Sumak
Sp. Zumaque
It. Sommacco
Gr. Roúdhi; Soumáki
Gr. Ρούδι· Σουμάκι
H. Szömörce
P. Sumak
T. Sumak

604. *Ribes nigrum*
E. Blackcurrant
F. Cassis
G. Schwarze Johannisbeere
S. Svarta vinbär
Sp. Grosellero negro
It. Ribes nero
Gr. Mávro frangostáphylo
Gr. Μαύρο
φραγκοστάφυλο
H. Fekete ribiszke
P. Porzeczka czarna
T. Frenk üzümü

605. *Ribes rubrum*
E. Redcurrant
F. Groseille
G. Rote Johannisbeere
S. Trägårdsvinbär
Sp. Grosellero
It. Ribes rosso
Gr. Frangostáphyllo
Gr. Φραγκοστάφυλο
H. Piros ribiszke
P. Porzeczka czerwona
T. Kırmızı frenk
üzümü

606. *Ribes uva-crispa*
E. Gooseberry
F. Groseille à maquereau;
G. Stachelbeere
S. Krusbär
Sp. Grosello espinosa
It. Uva spina
Gr. Laghokéraso
Gr. Λαγοκέρασο
H. Egres
P. Agrest zółty
T. Bektaşi üzümü

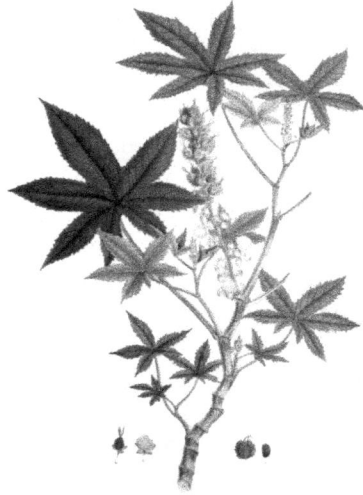

607. *Ricinus communis*
E. Castor-Oil Plant
F. Ricin
G. Rizinus pflanze
S. Ricin
Sp. Ricino común; Higuerilla
It. Ricino
Gr. Retsinoladhiá
Gr. Ρετσινολαδιά
H. Ricinus növény;
Csodafa
P. Rącznik; Ricynus
T. Hint yağı ağ.

608. *Rosa canina*
E. Dog Rose; Sweet Briar;
Rosehip
F. Églantine
G. Hundrose; Hagrose
S. Stenros
Sp. Rosa canina;
Escaranajo
It. Rosa canina
Gr. Ághrio triandáfillo

Gr. Ἄγριο τριαντάφυλλο
H. Csipkebogyó; Csipkerózsa;
    Vad rózsa
P. Polna róża
T. Yabani gül; İt burnu

609. *Rosa spp.*
E. Rose
F. Rose
G. Rose
S. Ros
Sp. Rosa
It. Rosa
Gr. Triandáfillo; Ródho
Gr. Τριαντάφυλλο˙ Ρόδο
H. Rozsá
P. Róża
T. Gül

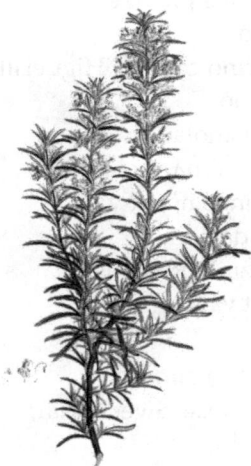

610. *Rosmarinus officinalis*
E. Rosemary
F. Romarin
G. Rosmarin
S. Rosmarin

Sp. Romero
It. Rosmarino
Gr. Dhendrolívano
Gr. Δενδρολίβανο
H. Rozmaring
P. Rozmaryn
T. Biberiye; Hasalban

611. *Rubia tinctorum*
E. Madder
F. Garance des teinturiers
G. Fäberröte; Krapp
S. Krapp
Sp. Rubia; Garanza
It. Robbia
Gr. Rizári; Aghrióvafion
Gr. Ριζάρι˙ Αγριόβαφιον
H. Festőbuzér
P. Marzana; Brocz
T. Kök boyası; Kızıl boya

612. *Rubus fructosus*
E. Blackberry
F. Mûre; Ronce des bois
G. Brombeere
S. Björnbär
Sp. Zarza; Mora; Frambuesa negra
It. Rovo
Gr. Vatómouro; Vátos
Gr. Βατόμουρο˙ Βάτος
H. Földi szeder
P. Jeżyna; Czernika
T. Böğürtlen çalısı

613. *Rubus idaeus*
E. Raspberry
F. Framboise
G. Himbeere
S. Hallon

Sp. Frambuesa
It. Lampone
Gr. Framboise; Sméouro
Gr. Φραμπουάζ· Σμέουρο
H. Málna
P. Malina
T. Ahu dudu

614. Rumex acetosa
E. Common Sorrel
F. Oseilles des prés
G. Sauer-Ampfer
S. Änggsyra
Sp. Acedera; Vinagrera
It. Acetosa; Erba brusca
Gr. Xiníthra; Xinolápatho
Gr. Ξινίθρα· Ξινολάπαθο
H. Sóska
P. Szczaw zwyczajny
T. Kuzu kulağı

615. Rumex acetosella
E. Sheep's Sorrel
F. Oseilles sauvage; Oseilles de
   brebis
G. Feld-Ampfer
S. Bergsyra
Sp. Acedera menor;
   Acederilla
It. Romice acetosella
Gr. Oxylápatho
Gr. Οξυλάπαθο
H. Juhsóska
P. Szczaw pospolity
T. Labada (küçük) kulağı

616. Rumex alpinus
E. Monk's Rhubarb; Patience
   Dock

F. Oseilles des Alpes; Patience
G. Alpen-Ampfer
S. Alpskräppa
Sp. Ruibarbo des monjes; Hierba
   paciencia
It. Lapazio; Erba pazienza
Gr. Lápathon; Roúmex o
   alpikós
Gr. Λάπαθον· Ρούμεξ ο
   αλπικός
H. Havasi lórem
P. Szczaw alpejski
T. Labadasi (dağ)

617. Rumex crispus
E. Yellow Dock
F. Rumex crépu
G. Krauser-Ampfer
S. Krusskräppa
Sp. Romaza crespa
It. Rumice crespo
Gr. Ághrio lápatho;
   Roúmex
Gr. Άγριο λάπαθο· Ρούμεξ
H. Fodros lórem
P. Szczaw kędzierzawy
T. Evelik

618. Ruscus aculeatus
E. Butcher's Broom
F. Petit-houx
G. Stechender Mäusedorn
S. Stickmyrten
Sp. Rusco
It. Rusco
Gr. Roúskos; Korallína;
   Laghomiliá
Gr. Ρούσκος· Κοραλίνα·
   Λαγομηλιά

H. Szúros csodabogyó
P. Myszopłoch; Grzbietolist
T. Ölmezdiken; Tavşanmemesi

619. Ruta graveolens
E. Rue
F. Rue
G. Raute; Weinraute
S. Vinruta
Sp. Ruta; Ruda
It. Ruta
Gr. Apíganos; Pígani
Gr. Απίγανος· Πίγανι
H. Ruta
P. Ruta
T. Sedef otu

620. Sabina vulgaris/Juniperus sabina
E. Savin; Savin Juniper
F. Sabine; Savinier
G. Sabinerbaum
S. Sävenbom
Sp. Sabina; Ginistra y groto romero
It. Sabina
Gr. Savína
Gr. Σαβίνα
H. Nehézszagú boróka
P. Jałowiec sawina
T. Ardıç (kara); Sabina ardıçı

621. Salicornia europaea
E. Glasswort; Marsh Samphire
F. Salicorne d'europe
G. Europäische Queller Glasschmalz
It. Salicornia erbacea

S. Glasört
Sp. Salicor
Gr. Salicórnia; Almiríki
Gr. Σαλικόρνια· Αλμιρίκι
H. Sziksófű; Sómócsing
P. Solirod zielny
T. Deniz börülcesi; Abu sak; Kurşun otu

622. Salix alba
E. White Willow
F. Saule Blanc
G. Silber Weide
S. Vitpil; Buskpil
Sp. Sauce blanco
It. Salice bianco
Gr. Itiá; Lefkí itiá
Gr. Ιτιά· Λευκή ιτιά
H. Fűz
P. Wierzba biała
T. Ak söğüt

623. Salsola kali
E. Saltwort
F. Soude; Salsolie
G. Gemeines Salzkraut
S. Sodaört
Sp. Barilla; Espinardo
It. Erba Kali
Gr. Sálsolo; Trivolón
Gr. Σάλσολο· Τριβολόν
H. Ballagófű
P. Solanka kolczysta
T. Üşnan; Döngele

T. Misk adaçayı

626. *Sambucus ebulus*
E. Dwarf Elder
F. Petit sureau; Yèble
G. Zwergholunder, Attich
S. Sommarfläder
Sp. Yezgo; Matapulgas
It. Ebbio; Sambuco lebbio
Gr. Vouziá
Gr. Βουζιά
H. Gyalag bodza
P. Bez hebd; Chabzina
T. Yaban mürverı; Yer mürverı

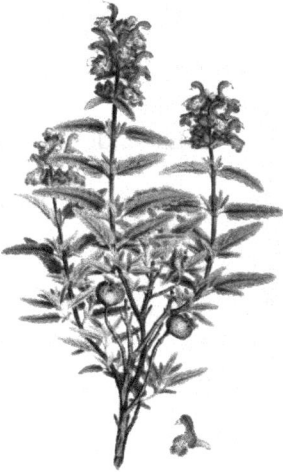

624. *Salvia officinalis*
E. Common Sage
F. Sauge
G. Salbei
S. Salvia; Kryddsalvia
Sp. Salvia
It. Salvia
Gr. Faskómilo
Gr. Φασκόμηλο
H. Zsálya
P. Szałwia
T. Adaçayı

627. *Sambucus nigra*
E. Elder
F. Sureau
G. Holunder
S. Fläder
Sp. Saúco; Sabugo
It. Sambuco
Gr. Zaboúkos; Koufoxiliá
Gr. Ζαμπούκος· Κουφοξυλιά
H. Bodza
P. Bez czarny
T. Kara Mürver ağ

625. *Salvia sclarea*
E. Clary Sage
F. Sauge sclarée
G. Muskateller Salbei
S. Muskatellsalvia
Sp. Esclarea; Amaro; Gallocresta
It. Salvia sclarea
Gr. Ayyánnis; Ghorghóyannis
Gr. Αϊγιάννης· Γοργογιάννης
H. Muskotályzsálya
P. Granatek

628. *Sanguinaria canadensis*
E. Bloodroot
F. Sanguinaire du Canada
G. Kanadische Blutwurz
S. Blodört
Sp. Sanguinaria
It. Sanguinaria
Gr. Ematóhorto
Gr. Αιματόχορτο
H. Véripipacs
P. Plewimaczek

T. Kankökü (Kanada)

629. Sanguisorbia officinalis
E. Greater Burnet
F. Sanguisorbe officinale
G. Grosser Wiesenknopf
S. Blodtopp
Sp. Pimpinela mayor
It. Salvastrella maggiore
Gr. Sangouisórba
Gr. Σανγουισόρμπα
H. Őszivérfű
P. Krwiściąg
T. Çayırdügmesi

630. Sanicula europaea
E. Sanicle
F. Sanicle
G. Sanikel
S. Sårläkor
Sp. Sanícula; Hierba de San
  Lorenzo
It. Sanicola; Erba Fragolina
Gr. Sanikoúla
Gr. Σανικούλα
H. Gombernyö
P. Zankiel
T. Deve kulağı; Sanikula

631. Santalum album
E. Sandalwood
F. Bois de santal
G. Sandelholz
S. Sandelträd
Sp. Sándalo
It. Sandalo
Gr. Sandhalóxylon
Gr. Σανδαλόξυλον
H. Szantálfa
P. Czyndalin; Sandałowe drzewo

T. Sandal ağacı

632. Santolina chamaecyparissus
E. Santolina; Lavender Cotton
F. Santoline
G. Heiligenkraut, Graues;
  Buchzypress
S. Grå helgonört
Sp. Abrótano hembra
It. Santolina
Gr. Santolíni
Gr. Σαντολίνη
H. Cipruska
P. Świętolina
T. Lavantin

633. Saponaria officinalis
E. Soapwort
F. Saponaire; Savonnière
G. Gemeines Seifenkraut
S. Såpnejlika
Sp. Saponaria; Hierba jabonera
It. Saponaria
Gr. Sapounóhorto
Gr. Σαπουνόχορτο
H. Szappanfű
P. Mydlnica
T. Sabun otu

634. Sargassum fussiform
E. Gulfweed
F. Sargasse
G. Sargassum
Sp. Sargazo bacifero
It. Uva di mare
Gr. Sárghasso
Gr. Σάργασσο
H. Tengeri hínár
P. Morzypło

635. *Sassafras officinalis*
E. Sassafras
F. Sassafras
G. Sassafras
S. Sassafras
Sp. Sasafrás
It. Sassofrasso
Gr. Sassafrás
Gr. Σασσαφράς
H. Szaszafrász
P. Sasafras
T. Sasafras

636. *Satureja hortensis*
E. Summer Savory
F. Sarriette des jardins
G. Sommer Bohnenkraut
S. Sommarkyndel
Sp. Ajedrea de jardin; Jedrea
It. Santoreggia domestica; Cerea
Gr. Throúmbi; Satouréia
Gr. Θρούμπη· Σατουρέϊα
H. Csombor
P. Cząber ogrodowy
T. Geyik otu; Sa'ter otu

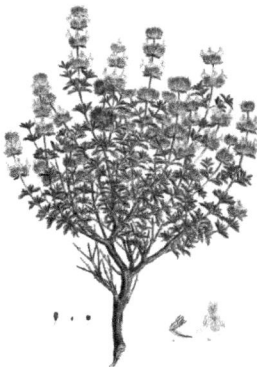

637. *Satureja montana*
E. Winter Savory

F. Sariette des montagnes
G. Winter Bohnenkraut
S. Vinterkyndel
Sp. Ajedrea; Hispillo
It. Santoreggia montana;
    Cerea
Gr. Throúmbi tou vounoú
Gr. Θρούμπη του βουνού
H. Borsfű
P. Cząber górski
T. Dağ sateri

638. *Scabiosa succisa*
E. Devil's Bit Scabious
F. Scabieuse des prés
G. Hängeweide
S. Ängsvädd
Sp. Freno del diablo
It. Vedovina dei prati
Gr. Stourakiá;
    Astírakas
Gr. Στουρακιά· Αστήρακας
H. Ördögszem
P. Drakiew
T. Uyuz otu

639. *Scrophularia nodosa*
E. Figwort
F. Scrophulaire nodeuse
G. Knotige Braunwurz
S. Flenört
Sp. Escrofularia; Hierba de
    lamparones
It. Scrofularia nodosa; Mille
    morbia
Gr. Skrofoulária
Gr. Σκροφουλάρια
H. Görvélfű
P. Trędownik
T. Sıraca otu

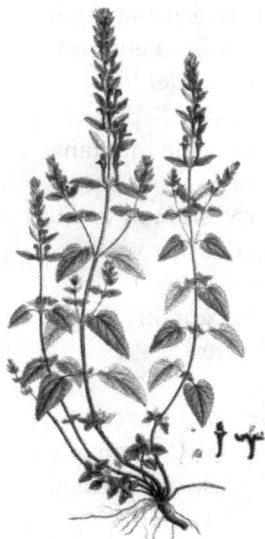

640. Scutellaria laterifolia
E. Skullcap
F. Scutellaire; Toque casquée
G. Sumpfhelmkraut
S. Frossört
Sp. Tercianaria; Craneo
It. Scutellaria
Gr. Skoutellária
Gr. Σκουτελάρια
H. Vízmelléki csukóko
P. Tarczyca
T. Kaside otu

641. Secale cereale
E. Rye
F. Siegle
G. Roggen
S. Råg
Sp. Centeno
It. Segale
Gr. Síkali
Gr. Σίκαλη

H. Rozs
P. Żyto
T. Çavdar

642. Sedum acre
E. Biting Stonecrop; Wall-pepper
F. Orpin âcre; Poivre des
     murailles; Sedum âcre
G. Scharfer Mauerpfeffer
S. Gul fetknopp
Sp. Pampajarito
It. Erba pignola; Pepe dei muri
Gr. Kohilóhorto; Petróhorto
Gr. Κοχυλόχορτο˙ Πετρόχορτο
H. Varjúhaj
P. Pryszczyrnik; Rozczodnik
T. Acı dam koruğu

643. Selenicereus grandiflora
E. Night Blooming Cactus
F. Cactier
G. Kaktus
S. Kaktus
Sp. Cactus
It. Cacto
Gr. Káktos
Gr. Κάκτος
H. Kaktusz
P. Kaktus
T. Kaktüs

644. Sempervivum tectorum
E. Houseleek
F. Joujarbe des toits
G. Hauswurz; Dachwurz
S. Taklök
Sp. Siempreviva mayor; Hierba
     puntera
It. Porro sempreviva

Gr. Sebervívo to epístegho
Gr. Σεμπερβίβο το επίστεγο
H. Kövirózsa; Fűlfu
P. Rojnik; Skoczek
T. Dam koruğu; Kulakotu

645. Senecio jacobea
E. Ragwort
F. Séneçon jacobée
G. Jakobskraut
S. Stånds
Sp. Hierba de Santiago; Zuson
It. Erba di San Giacomo; Erba
    Chitarra
Gr. Senétsio
Gr. Σενέτσιο
H. Aggófű; Szent Jákob fűve
P. Starzec jakubek
T. Yakub otu

646. Senecio vulgaris
E. Groundsel
F. Séneçon commun
G. Gemeines Kreuzkraut
S. Korsört
Sp. Hierba cana
It. Calderugia; Senecio
Gr. Martiákos
Gr. Μαρτιάκος
H. Aggkóro; Aggófu
P. Starzec pospolity; Kryżownik
T. Kanarya otu

647. Serenoa serrulata
E. Saw Palmetto
F. Sabal; Chou palmiste
G. Sägepalme
S. Sågpalmetto
Sp. Sabal
It. Sabal

Gr. Sabál; Serenóa
Gr. Σαμπάλ˙ Σερενόα
H. Fűrészpálma
P. Palma karlowata
T. Cűce palmiye

648. Sesamum indicum
E. Sesame
F. Sésame
G. Sesam
S. Sesam
Sp. Sésamo; Ajonjol
It. Sesamo
Gr. Sousámi
Gr. Σουσάμι
H. Szezámmag
P. Sezam
T. Susam

649. Silybum marianum
E. Milk Thistle
F. Chardon Marie
G. Mariendistel
S. Mariatistel
Sp. Cardo Maria
It. Cardo Mariano
Gr. Gaïdhourágatho
Gr. Γαϊδουράγκαθο
H. Máriatövis
P. Ostropest plamisty;
    Pstrost
T. Devedikeni; Meryemana dikeni

650. Simmondsia chinensis
E. Jojoba
F. Jojoba
G. Jojoba
S. Jojoba
Sp. Jojoba
It. Jojoba

Gr. Jojoba
Gr. Χοχόμπα
H. Jojoba
P. Jojoba

651. Sinapis alba→
Brassica alba

652. Sinapis arvensis→
Brassica sinapistrum

653. Sinapis nigra→
Brassica nigra

654. Sisymbrium officinale
E. Hedge Mustard
F. Herbe aux chantres; Vélar
G. Wegrauke
S. Vägsenap
Sp. Erismo officinal
It. Erismo; Erba dei cantanti
Gr. Sisímbrio to farmakeftikón
Gr. Σισίμπριο το
    φαρμακευτικόν
H. Szapora zsombor
P. Stulisz; Rukiew
T. Ergelen hardalı

655. Smilax officinalis
E. Sarsaparilla
F. Salseparille; Smilax
G. Sarsaparille; Stechwinde
S. Sarsaparille
Sp. Zarzaparilla
It. Salsapariglia; Smilace
Gr. Smílax
Gr. Σμίλαξ
H. Saszaparilla
P. Sarsaparylla; Kolcowój

T. Saparnası (Jamaika); Silcan otu

656. Smyrnium olusatrum
E. Alexanders; Black Lovage
F. Maceron
G. Pferdeeppich
S. Alexanderloka
Sp. Apio caballar; Esmirnio
It. Macerone
Gr. Mávro sélino; Pikrostafidha
Gr. Μαύρο σέλινο·
    Πικροσταφίδα
H. Őzsaláta; Lópetrezselyem
P. Gierszownik
T. Yabani kereviz; Deli kereviz

657. Solanum carolinense
E. Horsenettle
F. Morelle aviculaire
G. Carolina-Nachtschatten
Sp. Poroporo; Uva de perro
It. Morella della
    Carolina
Gr. Solanó Karolínas
Gr. Σολανό Καρολίνας

658. Solanum dulcamare
E. Woody Nightshade;
    Bittersweet
F. Douce- amère
G. Bittersüsser Nachtschatten
S. Besksöta
Sp. Dulcarama; Amardulce; Uva
    del Diablo
It. Dulcamare
Gr. Strignós; Aghióklima
Gr. Στριγκνός· Αγιόκλιμα
H. Piros ebszőlő; Édes keserű
    csucsor

P. Psianka słodkogórz;
Rzemieniec
T. Yabancı yasemini; Sofur

659. *Solanum melongena*
E. Aubergine; Eggplant
F. Aubergine
G. Aubergine; Eierfrucht
S. Aubergin
Sp. Berenjena
It. Melanzana
Gr. Melinzána
Gr. Μελινζάνα
H. Padlizsán
P. Bakłażan
T. Patlican; Batincan

660. *Solanum nigrum*
E. Black Nightshade
F. Morelle noir
G. Schwarzer Nachtschatten
S. Nattskatta
Sp. Hierba mora; Tomatillos del
diablo
It. Erba morella; Solano nero
Gr. Stífno; Mavróhorto
Gr. Στίφνο˙ Μαυρόχορτο
H. Fekete csucsor
P. Psianka csarna
T. Köpek üzümü; Sofur (kara)

661. *Solanum tuberosum*
E. Potatoe
F. Pomme de terre
G. Kartoffel
S. Potatis
Sp. Patata; Papa
It. Patata
Gr. Patáta

Gr. Πατάτα
H. Burgonya
P. Kartofel; Ziemniak
T. Patates

662. *Solidago virguarea*
E. Golden Rod; Aaron's Rod
F. Solidage; Verge d'or
G. Echte Goldrute
S. Gullris
Sp. Vara de oro
It. Verga d'oro
Gr. Solidhágo; Chrisóverga
Gr. Σολιδάγκο˙ Χρυσόβεργα
H. Aranyvessző
P. Nawłoć; Złota rózga
T. Adi altınbaşak;
Altınbaşak otu

663. *Sonchus oleraceus*
E. Common Sow Thistle
F. Laiteron potager
G. Gänsedistel
S. Kålmolke
Sp. Cerraja; Lechecino
It. Crespino; Cicerbita
Gr. Zohós
Gr. Ζοχός
H. Mezei csoborka
P. Mlécz warzywny
T. Eşek marulu; Hassi kiazib

664. *Sorbus aucuparia*
E. Rowan; Mountain Ash
F. Sorbier des oiseleurs; Sorbier
sauvage
G. Vogelbeerbaum; Gemeine
Eberesche
S. Rönn

Sp. Serbal
It. Sorbo degli uccelli
Gr. Sórbous, sourviá
Gr. Σόρμπους
H. Berkenye
P. Jarząb
T. Yabani üvez ağ.; Kuş üvesi

665. Spartium junceum
E. Spanish Broom
F. Gênet d'Espagne; Ginistre spartier
G. Bisenginster; Spanischer Ginster
S. Spanskginst
Sp. Gayomba; Retama de olor
It. Ginestra di Spagna
Gr. Spártio
Gr. Σπάρτιο
H. Spanyol rekettye
P. Szczodrzenica sitowata
T. Süpürgı katırtırnağı

666. Sphagnum cimbilifolium
E. Sphagnum Moss; Bog Moss
F. Sphaigne
G. Torfmoos
S. Trubb-vitmossa
Sp. Musgo esfagno
It. Muschio di palude
Gr. Vríon; Moúsklo
Gr. Βρύον˙ Μούσκλο
H. Tőzegmoha
P. Torfowiec
T. Yosun; Ketencik

667. Spigelia marilandica
E. Pinkroot
F. Spigélie anthelmique

G. Wurmkraut
S. Spigelia
Sp. Spigelia
It. Spigelia; Erba da bachi
Gr. Spigélia i marilandhikí
Gr. Σπιγκέλια η μαριλανδική
H. Tüzes szegfűgyökér
P. Czerwioda

668. Spinacea oleracea
E. Spinach
F. Épinard
G. Spinat
S. Spenat
Sp. Espinaca
It. Spinaci
Gr. Spanáki
Gr. Σπανάκι
H. Spenót; Paraj
P. Szpinak
T. İspanak

669. Stachys betonica→ Betonica officinalis

670. Stachys palustris
E. Marsh Woundwort
F. Epiaire des marais; Ortie morte
G. Sumpfziest
S. Knölsyska
Sp. Betónica palustre
It. Spigo fiorito; Streghona palustre
Gr. Stáchys o eloharís
Gr. Στάχυς ο ελοχαρίς
H. Mocsári tisztesfű
P. Cześciec błotny
T. Gölısırganı

671. Stachys sylvatica
E. Hedge Woundwort
F. Epiaire des bois; Ortie puante
G. Waldziest
S. Stinksyska
Sp. Ortiga hedionda
It. Matricale, Stregona dei boschi;
Erba giudaica
Gr. Stáchys o dhasikós
Gr. Στάχυς ο δασικός
H. Erdei tisztesfű
P. Cząciec leśny
T. Hamısırgan

672. Statice carolinianum
E. Sea Lavender
F. Lavande de mer
G. Echter Widerstoss
S. Strandrisp
It. Statice maritimo; Butolo
d'acqua
Gr. Limonio karolinas
Gr. Λιμώνειο καρολίνας
H. Tengerparti sóvirág
P. Zatrwien
T. Deniz lavantası

673. Stellaria media
E. Chickweed
F. Mouron des oiseaux;
Stellaire
G. Vogelmiere
S. Våtarv
Sp. Alsine; Pamplina
It. Centocchio; Paparina;
Mordigallina
Gr. Stellária
Gr. Στελάρια
H. Tyúkhúr

P. Muchotrzew; Gwiazdnica
T. Kusotu

674. Stillingia sylvatica
E. Queen's Delight; Yaw Root
F. Stillingie
G. Stillingie
S. Stillingia
It. Albero del sego
Gr. Stillígia
Gr. Στιλίγκια

675. Strophanthus hispidus
E. Strophanthus
F. Strophante
G. Strophantus
S. Strofant
Sp. Strofanto
It. Strofanto
Gr. Strofantós
Gr. Στροφαντός
H. Szenegáli selyemperje
P. Strofant

676. Strychnos nux-vomica
E. Nux Vomica; Poison Nut
F. Vomique noix
G. Brechnuss
S. Rävkaketräd
Sp. Nuez vomica
It. Noce vomica
Gr. Strýchnos o emetikós
Gr. Στρίχνος ο εμετικός
H. Farkasmaszlag
P. Kulczyba
T. Karga büken ağ.

677. Styrax benzoin
E. Benzoin

F. Benjoin
G. Styraxstrauch
S. Bensoeträd
Sp. Bálsamo de benjuí; Bejul
It. Benzoino
Gr. Venzói
Gr. Βενζόη
H. Benzoégyanta
P. Benzoes
T. Azılbend; Kara günlük ağ

678. Styrax officinalis→
Liquidamber orientalis

679. Succharum officinarum
E. Sugar Cane
F. Canne à sucre
G. Zuckerrohr
S. Sockerrör
Sp. Caña de azúcar
It. Canna da zucchero
Gr. Zacharokálamo
Gr. Ζαχαροκάλαμο
H. Cukornád
P. Trzcina cukrowa
T. Şeker kamışı

680. Swertia chirata
E. Chiretta; Indian
    Gentian
F. Swertie
G. Ostindischer-Enzian
S. Chirette
Sp. Ciretta
It. Chiretta; Swertia
Gr. Kiréta; Souértia
Gr. Κιρέτα˙ Σουέρτια;
H. Indiai gyásztárnics
P. Niebielistka chiretta
T. Svertia

681. Symphytum officinalis
E. Comfrey
F. Consoude
G. Schwarzwurz;
    Beinwell
S. Vallört
Sp. Consuelda mayor
It. Consolida maggiore;
    Sinfito
Gr. Stekoúli; Sýmphyto; Aftí tou
    ghaïdhárou
Gr. Στεκούλι˙ Σύμφυτο˙ Αυτί
    του γαϊδάρου
H. Nadálytő
P. Żywokost
T. Karakafes otu

682. Symplocarpus foetidus
E. Skunk-Cabbage
F. Symplocarpe
G. Stinkkohl
S. Fläckig skunkkalla
Sp. Repollo oloroso
It. Draconzio
Gr. Symplókarpos i dhísosmos
Gr. Συμπλόκαρπος η
    δύσοσμος
H. Büdös kontyvirág
P. Skypnia cuchnąca

683. Syringa vulgaris
E. Lilac
F. Lilas
G. Flieder
S. Syren
Sp. Lilo
It. Lillá; Serenella
Gr. Paschaliá
Gr. Πασχαλιά
H. Orgona; Lila

P. Lilak
T. Leylak

684. *Syzygium aromaticum*→
Eugenia caryophyllus

685. *Tagetes patula*
E. French Marigold; Tagetes
F. Tagète; Veloutine; Œillet
   d'Inde
G. Sammtblume
S. Sammetsblomster
Sp. Cepetillo; Mercadela
It. Tagete
Gr. Taghétis
Gr. Ταγέτις
H. Büdöske
P. Aksamitka
T. Kadife çiçeği

686. *Tamarindus indica*
E. Tamarind
F. Tamarin; Tamarinde
G. Tamarinde
S. Tamarind
Sp. Tamarindo
It. Tamarindo
Gr. Tamaríndo
Gr. Ταμαρίντο
H. Tamarindusz
P. Tamaryndowiec
T. Temir hindi; Hint hurması

687. *Tamarix mannifera*
E. Manna Tamarix
F. Tamaris à manne
G. Tamarisk Manna
S. Manna tamarisk
Sp. Tamarisco de manna
It. Tamarice di manna

Gr. Armiríki
Gr. Αρμυρίκι
H. Mannacserje
P. Września manna; Tamaryszek
   manna
T. Manna ılgun ağ.

688. *Tamus communis*
E. Black Bryony
F. Tarnier commun; Herbes aux
   femmes battues
G. Schmerzwurz
S. Djävulsdruva
Sp. Brionia; Canduerca
It. Tamaro; Vite nera
Gr. Vrionía; Avrónia;
   Ovriá
Gr. Βριονία˙ Αβρόνια˙ Οβριά
H. Közönséges pirítógyökér
P. Przelaj
T. Siyah akasma; Dövülmüs
   avratotu

689. *Tanacetum balsamita*
E. Alecost; Costmary
F. Balsamite; Tanaisie grande
G. Marienblatt; Balsamit
S. Balsamblad
Sp. Balsamita
It. Barbotino
Gr. Karyophýlli; Tanatséto
   válsamo
Gr. Καρυοφύλλι; Τανατσέτο
   βάλσαμο
H. Balszamita
P. Wrotycz szerokolistny
T. Marsuvan otu

690. *Tanacetum cinerarifolium*
E. Pyrethrum

F. Pyrèthre
G. Dalmatinische Insektenblume
S. Dalmatinerkrage
Sp. Pelitre
It. Piretro
Gr. Pýrethron
Gr. Πύρεθρον
H. Morzsika
P. Złocień dalmatiński
T. Dalmaçya pire otu

691. Tanacetum parthenium
E. Feverfew
F. Partenelle; Grande camomille
G. Mutterkraut
S. Mattram
Sp. Boton de plata; Matricara
It. Crisantemo partenio;
Amareggiola; Matricaleσσ
Gr. Parthenoúli; Vaskadhíra
Gr. Παρθενούλι· Βασκαδίρα
H. Öszi margitvirág
P. Wrotycz maruna
T. Gümüşdüğme

692. Tanacetum vulgare
E. Tansy
F. Tanaisie; Barbotine; Set-bon
G. Rainfarn
S. Renfana
Sp. Tanaceto; Santa Maria;
Atanasia
It. Tanaceto; Atanasia
Gr. Tanatséto; Tanákiton;
Athánaton
Gr. Τανατσέτο· Τανάκητον·
Αθάνατον
H. Baradicskóró
P. Wrotycz pospolity

T. Solucan otu

693. Taraxacum officinale
E. Dandelion
F. Pissenlit; Dent de lion
G. Löwenzahn; Kuhblume
S. Maskros; Sallatsmaskros
Sp. Diente de león; Amargon
It. Dente di leone; Radichiella;
Tarassaco
Gr. Taráxakon; Aghrio radhíki;
Pikralídha
Gr. Ταράξάκον· Άγριο ραδίκι·
Πικραλίδα
H. Pitypang;
Gyermekláncfu
P. Mniszek
T. Kara hindiba; Aslan dişi;
Yabani acı marul

694. Taxus baccata
E. Yew
F. If
G. Eibe
S. Idegran
Sp. Tejo
It. Tasso
Gr. Táxos
Gr. Τάξος
H. Tiszafa
P. Cis
T. Porsuk ağ.

695. Teucrium chamaedrys
E. Wall Germander
F. Germandrée petit chêne
G. Gemeiner Gamander
S. Gamander
Sp. Camedrio; Germandria

It. Camedrio
Gr. Téfkrion; Hamaedhrís
Gr. Τεύκριον˙ Χαμεδρίς
H. Gamandor
P. Ożanka
T. Kemedris; Dalak otu;
  Kısamahmut otu

S. Lundgamander
Sp. Escorodonia
It. Scordio; Erba aglio;
  Polio montana
Gr. Skordhéo
Gr. Σκορδέο
H. Zsályagamandor
P. Czosnak

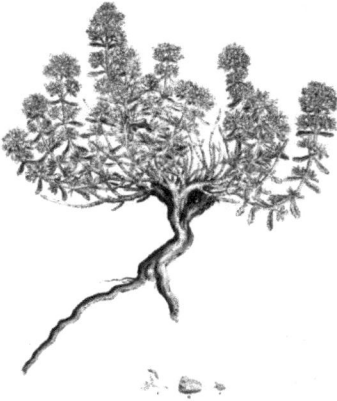

696. *Teucrium polium*
E. Felty Germander
F. Polium; Germandrée
  tomenteuse
G. Polei-Gamander
S. Buskgamander
Sp. Zamarrilla; Poleo del monte
It. Camedrio polio; Canutola
Gr. Laghokimisiá
Gr. Λαγοκοιμησιά
H. Rozmaring-gamandor
P. Polej; Siwiosnka
T. Acıyavşan

697. *Teucrium scorodonia*
E. Wood Sage
F. Germandrée des bois
G. Salbei-Gamander

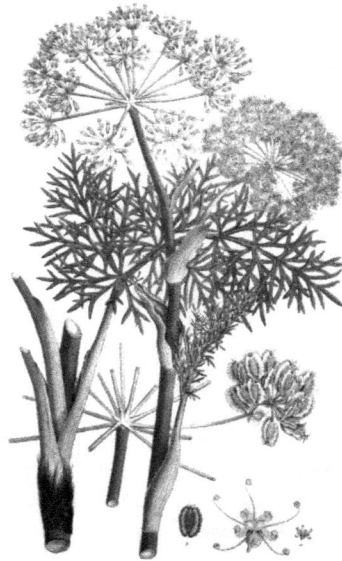

698. *Thapsia garganica*
E. Deadly Carrot; Drias
F. Thapsie; Turbith;
  Faux fenouil
G. Böskraut; Falsche Turbith
S. Gulrot
Sp. Tapsia
It. Tapsia; Turbitto di Puglia
Gr. Thápsia; Polýkarpos
Gr. Θάψια˙ Πολύκαρπος
P. Trzcian
T. Delikörek

699. *Theobroma cacao*

E. Cocoa
F. Cacao
G. Kakao
S. Kakao
Sp. Cacao
It. Cacao
Gr. Kakáo
Gr. Κακάο
H. Kakaó
P. Kakaowiec
T. Kakao

700. *Thuja occidentalis*

E. Thuja; Arbor-Vitae
F. Thuya
G. Lebensbaum
S. Tuja
Sp. Arbol de la vida
It. Tuja
Gr. Toúiya
Gr. Τούια
H. Tuja; Életfa;
   Arbor-vitae
P. Żywotnik
T. Batı mazısı

701. *Thymus serpyllum*

E. Wild Thyme; Serpyllum
F. Serpolet; Thym sauvage
G. Sandthymian
S. Backtimjan
Sp. Serpol; Tomillo
   silvestre
It. Timio serpillo
Gr. Thymári
Gr. Θυμάρι
H. Mezei kakukkfű
P. Maczierzanka
T. Kekik (yabani)

702. *Thymus vulgaris*

E. Common Thyme
F. Thym cultivé
G. Gartenthymian; Kuttelkraut
S. Kryddtimjan
Sp. Tomillo
It. Timio volgare
Gr. Thymári
Gr. Θυμάρι
H. Kakukkfű
P. Tymianek
T. Kekik; Hakiki kekik; Bahçe
   kekiği

703. *Tilia europaea*

E. Lime Tree; Linden Flowers
F. Tilleul
G. Linden
S. Lind
Sp. Tilo
It. Tilgio
Gr. Tílio; Flamouriá
Gr. Τίλιο· Φλαμουριά
H. Harsfa
P. Lipa; Lipina
T. Ihlamur

704. *Tragopogon porrifolius*

E. Salsify; Vegetable Oyster
F. Salsifis
G. Haferwurzel
S. Äkta haverrot
Sp. Salsifi
It. Scorzonera
Gr. Traghopóghon; Lagóhorto
Gr. Τραγοπώγων· Λαγόχορτο
H. Közönséges bakszakáll
P. Salsefia; Kozibród porolistny
T. İskorçina; Tekesakalı çiçeği;
   Yemlik

705. *Tragopogon pratensis*
E. Goat's Beard; Moonflower
F. Barbe de bouc; Salsifis
  sauvage
G. Weisenbockbart
S. Ängshaverrot
Sp. Barba cabruna; Barbón
It. Barba di becco
Gr. Ghénya tou laghoú
Gr. Γένια του λαγού
H. Réti Bakszakáll
P. Kosibród łąkowy; Wliśnik
T. Salsifin; Sarı salsifin

706. *Trifolium pratensis*
E. Red Clover
F. Trèfle des prés
G. Rotklee
S. Rödklöver
Sp. Trébol rojo; Carreton
  morado
It. Trifoglio rosso
Gr. Kókkino trifíli
Gr. Κόκκινο τριφύλλι
H. Bíbor lóhere
P. Koniczyna łąkowa
T. Üç kulak otu; Kırmızı yonca

707. *Triglochin maritima*
E. Sea Arrow-Grass
F. Troscart maritime
G. Meerstranddreizack
S. Havssälting
Sp. Junco bastardo marino
It. Gincastrello marino
Gr. Trighlóchlin o parálios
Gr. Τριγλώχλιν ο
  παράλιος
H. Tengerparti kígyófű
P. Świebka; Błotnica

708. *Trigonella foenum-graecum*
E. Fenugreek
F. Fenugrec; Trigonelle
G. Bockshornklee
S. Bockhornsklöver
Sp. Alholva; Fenogreco
It. Fieno greco
Gr. Trighonélla; Tsiméni;
  Nicháki
Gr. Τριγωνέλλα· Τσιμένι·
  Νυχάκι
Ar. Hhulbah; Hhelbah
H. Görögszena
P. Kozieradka; Boża trawka
T. Çemen otu

709. *Trillium erectum*
E. Bethroot; Birthroot
F. Trille dressé
G. Dreiblatt
S. Purpurtreblad
Gr. Tríllio
Gr. Τρίλλιο
H. Vörösbarna
  hármasszirom
P. Trzypotrzyca; Trojak

**710. *Triticum repens*→
*Agropyrens repens***

711. *Triticum vulgare*
E. Wheat
F. Blé
G. Weizen
S. Vete
Sp. Trigo
It. Grano
Gr. Sitári
Gr. Σιτάρι

H. Búza
P. Pszenica
T. Buğday

712. Tropaeolum majus
E. Nasturtium
F. Capucine grande
G. Kapuziner Kresse
S. Indiankrasse
Sp. Capuchina
It. Cappuccina; Nasturzio
  indiano
Gr. Nástourtion; Nerokárdhamo
Gr. Ναστούρτιον˙ Νεροκάρδαμο
H. Sarkantyúvirág
P. Nasturcja
T. Latin çiç

713. Tuber melenosporum
E. Truffle
F. Truffe
G. Schwarze Trüffel
S. Svart tryffel
Sp. Trufa
It. Tartufo
Gr. Troúffa
Gr. Τρούφα
H. Szarvasgomba
P. Trufla
T. Yer mantarı; Trűf mantarı

714. Turnera diffusa
E. Damiana
F. Damiana; Bourrique
G. Damiana
S. Damiana
Sp. Damiana
It. Damiana
Gr. Damiána; Tournéria
Gr. Νταμιάνα˙ Τουρνέρια

H. Damiána
T. Damiana

715. Tussilago farfara
E. Coltsfoot
F. Tussilage; Pas d'âne
G. Huflattich
S. Hästhov
Sp. Tusilago; Pie de cavallo
It. Farfara; Piede d'asino;
  Tossilagine
Gr. Víxio; Tousilágo; Hamoléfki
Gr. Βίξιο˙ Τουσιλάγκο˙
  Χαμολεύκη
H. Martilapu; Szattyú
P. Podbiał
T. Öksürük otu; Kabalak otu;
  Farfara otu

716. Typha latifolia
E. Cat's Tail; Great Reedmace
F. Grande massette
G. Grosser Rohrkolben
S. Bredkaveldun
Sp. Anea; Espadaña
It. Mazzasorda; Tifa
Gr. Kalamiá
Gr. Καλαμιά
H. Nádbuzogany
P. Palka szerokolistna; Rogoża
T. Hasır otu; Su kamışı

717. Ulex europaeas
E. Gorse
F. Ajonc
G. Stechginster
S. Ättörne
Sp. Tojo; Retama espinosa
It. Ginestrone
Gr. Ráchos

Gr. Ράχος
H. Sünzanót, sülbige
P. Kolcolist; Złotochróst
T. Katır tırnağı

718. *Ulmus fulva/rubra*
E. Slippery Elm
F. Orme rousse; Orme rouge
G. Rot Ulme
S. Rödalm
Sp. Olmo babosa
It. Olmo rossa
Gr. Pteléa i amerikanikí
Gr. Πτελέα η αμερικανική
H. Vörös szil, Szilfakéreg
P. Wiąz czerwony
T. Kaygan karaağaç

719. *Ulmus vulgaris*
E. Elm
F. Orme
G. Ulme
S. Alm
Sp. Olmo
It. Olmo
Gr. Fteliá; Pteléa
Gr. Φτελιά; Πτελέα
H. Szil
P. Wiąz
T. Kara ağ.

720. *Umbilicus rupestris*
E. Pennywort; Navelwort
F. Écuelle; Nombril-de-Venus
G. Nabelkraut
S. Navelört
Sp. Ombligo de Venus
It. Ombelico di Venere
Gr. Oubílikos o vrachófilos
Gr. Ουμπίλικος ο βραχόφιλος

H. Köldökvirág
P. Urocznik; Pępek i pępownica
T. Göbekotu; Yuvarlak yapraklı bitki

721. *Uncaria tomentosa*
E. Cat's Claw
F. Uncaria
G. Katzenkralle
S. Cat's claw
Sp. Uña de gato
It. Uncaria
Gr. Ounkária i trichotí
Gr. Ουνκάρια η τριχωτί
P. Czepota
T. Kedi pençesi otu

722. *Urginea maritima*
E. Sea Squill
F. Ognion maritime; Scille
    maritime
G. Meerzwiebel
S. Sjölök
Sp. Escila
It. Scilla maritima
Gr. Skílla; Kromídha; Koutsoúpa
Gr. Σκίλλα· Κρομμίδα·
    Κουτσούπα
H. Tengeri csillagvirág
P. Oszloch; Cebula morska
T. Ada soğanı; Kum örümcekotu

723. *Urtica dioica*
E. Nettle; stinging
F. Ortie
G. Nessel
S. Brännässla
Sp. Ortiga
It. Ortica
Gr. Tsouknídha
Gr. Τσουκνίδα

H. Csalán
P. Pokrzywa; Żegawka
T. Isırğan otu

724. Usnea barbata
E. Old Man's Beard; Usnea
F. Usnée barbue; Barbe de
capucin
G. Bartflechten
S. Skägglav
Sp. Barba de capuchino
It. Lichene fiorito
Gr. Ghénya elátou;
Dhendhromaliá
Gr. Γένια ελάτου· Δενδρομαλιά
H. Szakállas zuzmó
P. Brodaczka; Pakość
T. Sakal likeni; Sakal yogsunu

725. Vaccinium myrtillus
E. Bilberry; Blueberry;
Whortleberry
F. Myrtille
G. Heidelbeere; Blaubeere
S. Blåbär
Sp. Arándano; Mirtilo
It. Mirtillo
Gr. Mírtillon; Fíggi
Gr. Μίρτιλλον· Φίγγι
H. Fekete áfonya
P. Borówka czarna
T. Kırmızı ayı üzümü; Kızamık;
Çoban üzümü; Yaban mersini

726. Vaccinium oxycocos
E. Cranberry
F. Canneberge
G. Preiselbeere
S. Tranbär
Sp. Camarino

It. Moretta
Gr. Vakínio oxýkokkon
Gr. Βακκίνιο οξύκοκκον
H. Tözeg áfonya
P. Żurawina błotna
T. Ekşi-mor ağ.

727. Vaccinium vitis idaea
E. Cowberry
F. Airelle rouge
G. Kuhbeere
S. Lingon
Sp. Arándano rojo
It. Mirtillo rosso
Gr. Vátos i idaea
Gr. Βάτος η ιδαία
H. Piros áfonya
P. Borówka brusznica
T. Yaban mersini (Kırmızı);
Ayıçileği

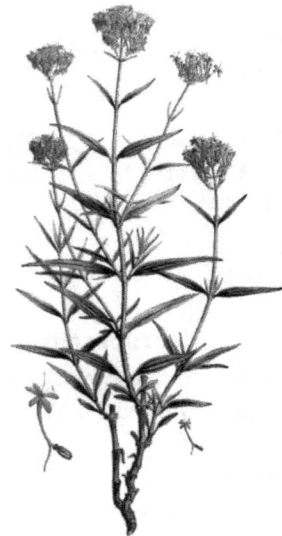

728. Valeriana officinalis
E. Valerian

F. Valériane; Herbe aux chats
G. Baldrian
S. Valeriana; Läkevänderot
Sp. Valeriana; Hierba de los gatos
It. Valeriana
Gr. Valeriána
Gr. Βαλεριάνα
H. Valerian; Macskagyökerfű
P. Bieldrzan; Kozłek lekarski
T. Kedi otu; Girit sümbülü

729. *Valerianella locusta*
E. Lamb's Lettuce
F. Mâche; Boursette
G. Ackersalat
S. Vårklynne
Sp. Dulceta; Hierba de los
  canónigos
It. Locusta; Gallinella
Gr. Valerianélla i topikí
Gr. Βαλεριανέλλα η τοπική
H. Galambbegy
P. Roszpunka warzywna; Sałatka
T. Nazlı; Kuzu kevreği

730. *Vanilla fragrens*
E. Vanilla
F. Vanille
G. Vanille
S. Vanilj
Sp. Vainilla
It. Vaniglia
Gr. Vanília
Gr. Βανίλια
H. Vanília
P. Wanilia
T. Vanilya

731. *Veratrum album*
E. White Hellebore

F. Verâtre blanc; Varaire
G. Weisser Germer
S. Nysrot
Sp. Verdegambre; Ballestera;
  Eléboro blanco
It. Elleboro bianco
Gr. Ellévoros i lefkí;
  Vératro
Gr. Ελλέβορος η λευκή·
  Βέρατρο
H. Fehér zászpa
P. Ciemiężyca biała
T. Dokuz tepeli; Kar çiç.

732. *Veratrum viride*→
Helleborus viridis

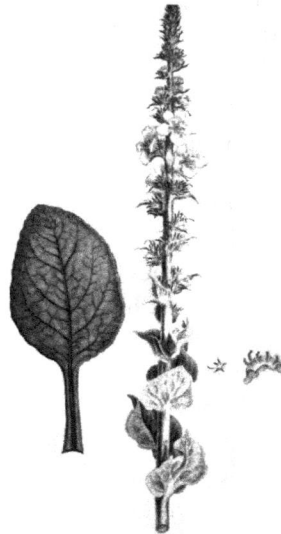

733. *Verbascum thapsus*
E. Mullein
F. Molène; Bouillon blanc
G. Königskerze
S. Kungsljus
Sp Gordolobo; Verbasco

It. Verbasco
Gr. Phlomós; Verbásko
Gr. Φλομός˙ Βερμπάσκο
H. Molyhos; Ökörfarkkóró
P. Dziewanna; Dziewizna
T. Sığir kuyruğu; Calba (kücük)

734. Verbena officinalis
E. Vervain
F. Verveine; Herbe sacrée
G. Eisenkraut
S. Järnört
Sp. Verbena; Hierba santa
It. Verbena
Gr. Vervéna; Stavróhorto;
    Yerovótano
Gr. Βερβένα˙ Σταυρόχορτο˙
    Γεροβότανο
H. Verbéna
P. Werbena; Witułka; Koszysko
T. Güvercin otu; Mine çiç.;
    Kanotu; Mineotu

735. Veronica beccabunga
E. Brooklime; Water Pimpernel
F. Cresson de cheval
G. Bachbungen Ehrenpreis
S. Bäckveronika
Sp. Verónica becabunga
It. Beccabunga
Gr. Avlakóhorto
Gr. Αυλακόχορτο
H. Deréceveronika
P. Przetacznik bobrowniczek
T. At teresi

736. Veronica officinalis
E. Speedwell
F. Veronique; Thé d'Europe
G. Ehrenpreis

S. Ärenpris
Sp. Verónica; Té de Europa
It. Tè svizzero
Gr. Veróniki
Gr. Βερόνικη
H. Orvosi Veronika
P. Przetacznik lesny
T. Yavsan otu; Çıban otu

737. Vetiveria zizanoides
E. Vetiver
F. Vétiver
G. Vetiver
S. Vetivergräs
Sp. Vetiver; Grama de la India
It. Vetivér
Gr. Vetivér
Gr. Βετιβέρ
H. Kuszkuszfű
P. Wetiweria
T. Vetiver

738. Viburnum opulus
E. Cramp Bark; Guelder Rose
F. Viorne obier; Écorce d'obier;
    Boule de neige
G. Gemeiner Schneeball
S. Skogsolvon
Sp. Bola de nieve; Mundillo; Rosa
    de quéldres
It. Viburno loppo
Gr. Vivoúrno to chionanthés
Gr. Βιβούρνο το χιονανθές
H. Labdarózsa
P. Kalina koralowa; Buldeneź
T. Gilaburu; Dağdığan ağ.

739. Viburnum prunifolium
E. Black Haw; Stagbush
F. Viorne; Viburnum

G. Pflaumenblättriger; Schneeball
S. Häggolvon
Sp. Viburno; Chuguaca
It. Viburno
Gr. Vivoúrno to prionófilon
Gr. Βιβούρνο το
πριονόφυλλον
H. Szilvalevelű bangita
P. Kalina śliwolistna

740. Vicia fava
E. Broad Bean
F. Fève
G. Saubohne
S. Bondböna
Sp. Habas
It. Fava
Gr. Koukkí
Gr. Κουκκί
H. Disznóbab
P. Bób
T. Bakla

741. Vinca major
E. Greater Periwinkle
F. Pervanche grande
G. Grosses Immergün
S. Stor vintergröna
Sp. Vincapervinca; Pervinca
major
It. Pervinca maggiore;
Mortine
Gr. Víga; Ághriolítsa
Gr. Βίγγα· Ἀγριολίτσα
H. Nagy meténg
P. Barwinek; Lubistek
T. Cezairmeneksesi

742. Vincitoxicum hirundinaria
E. Swallow-wort

F. Asclépiade blanche;
Dompte-venin
G. Schwalbenwurz
S. Tulkört
Sp. Matatósigo; Vencetósigo
It. Vincitossico
Gr. Alexitoxikón;
Asklipiádha
Gr. Ἀλεξιτοξικόν· Ἀσκλιπιάδα
H. Közönséges méreggyilok; Vad
paprika
P. Ciemiężyk białokwiatowy

743. Viola odorata
E. Sweet Violet
F. Violette odorante
G. Veilchen
S. Luktviol
Sp. Violeta
It. Violetta
Gr. Menexés; Violétta
Gr. Μενεξές· Βιολέττα
H. Ibolya
P. Fiołek
T. Menekşe; Benefşe

744. Viola tricolor
E. Heartease; Wild Pansy
F. Pensée sauvage
G. Dreifarbiges Veilchen; Wildes
Stiefmütterchen
S. Styvmorsviol
Sp. Pensamiento;
Trinitaria
It. Viola tricolor; Viola del
pensiero
Gr. Pánses; Víola
Gr. Πανσές· Βιόλα
H. Árvácska;
Császárszakáll

P. Fiołek trójbarwny;
  Brat
T. Hercayi menekşe

745. *Viscum album*
E. Mistletoe
F. Gui
G. Mistel
S. Mistel
Sp. Muérdago; Almuerdago
It. Vischio quercino
Gr. Ghí; Ixós
Gr. Γκί˙ Ιξός
H. Fagyöngy
P. Jemioła
T. Burç; Ökse otu; Gökce

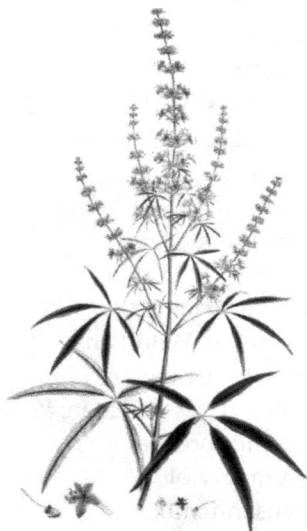

746. *Vitex agnus-castus*
E. Agnus castus; Vitex; Chaste
  Tree
F. Gattilier
G. Mönchspfeffer

S. Kyskhetsträd
Sp. Sauzgatillo; Pimiento loco;
  Hierba de San Josep
It. Agnocasto; Lagano
Gr. Lighariá
Gr. Λιγαριά
H. Szűzbariska; Szűzbokor
P. Niepokalanek
T. Hayıt

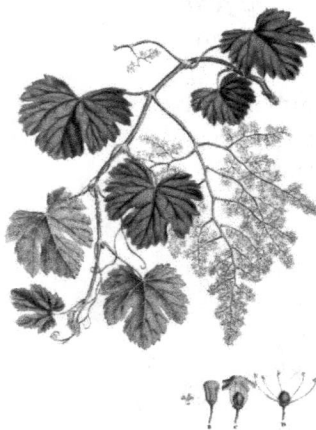

747. *Vitis vinifera*
E. Grapevine
F. Vigne
G. Weinstock
S. Vinranka
Sp. Vid
It. Vigna
Gr. Ábelos; Abelóklima
Gr. Ἄμπελος; Αμπελόκλιμα
H. Szőlőtő; Szőlővessző
P. Winorośl
T. Asma

747a. *Vitis vinifera*
E. Grape

F. Raisin
G. Traube
Sp. Uva
I. Uva
Gr. Stafíli
Gr. Σταφύλι
H. Szőlő
P. Winogrona
T. Üzüm

748. Withania somnifera

E. Winter Cherry; Ashwaghanda
F. Withanie
G. Winterkirsche; Ashwagandha
S. Withania; Indisk ginseng
Sp. Bufera somnifera; Oroval
It. Withania
Gr. Mertzánia
Gr. Μερζάνια
H. Álombogyó
T. Ashwagandha; Kış Kirazı

749. Xanthium spinosum

E. Spiny cocklebur; Prickly
  burweed
F. Lampourde épineuse
G. Dornige Spitzkette
S. Tistelgullfrö
Sp. Cachurera menor
It. Lappola spinosa
Gr. Xánthion
Gr. Ξάνθιον
H. Szúrós szerbtövis
P. Rzepien
T. Pıtrak; Hakiki sıraca otu

750. Yucca baccata

E. Yucca; Joshua Tree
F. Yucca

G. Yukka
S. Palmliljor
Sp. Yucca; Bayoneta
It. Yucca
Gr. Yúkka; Koróna
Gr. Γιούκα˙ Κορώνα
H. Jukka
P. Juka

751. Zanthoxylum americanum

E. Prickly Ash
F. Bois piquant; Fagarier
G. Zahnwehgelbholzbaum
S. Amerikanskt pepparträd
It. Ciava erculea
Gr. Xanthóxylon to
  amerikanikón
Gr. Ξανθόξυλον το
  αμερικανικόν
H. Amerikai sárgafa
P. Pieprz japoński
T. Dikenli diş budak ağ.

752. Zea mays

E. Corn
F. Maïs
G. Mais
S. Majs
Sp. Maíz
It. Granoturco; Mais
Gr. Kalambóki
Gr. Καλαμπόκι
H. Kukorica
P. Kukurydza; Kukuryza
T. Mısır

753. Zea mays

E. Cornsilk
F. Cheveux d'ange

G. Maiskolbenhaare
S. Majshår
Sp. Barba de maíz; Estilos de maíz
It. Barba granoturco
Gr. Maliá kalambokioú
Gr. Μαλλιά καλαμποκιού
H. Kukorica haj
P. Włosy kukurydzy
T. Mısır püşkülü

754. *Zingiber officinale*
E. Ginger
F. Gingembre
G. Ingwer
S. Ingfära
Sp. Gingibre; Jengibre
It. Zenzero
Gr. Tzitzer; Piperóriza

Gr. Ντζίντζερ· Πιπερόριζα
H. Gyömbér
P. Imbir
T. Zencefil; Zencebil

755. *Ziziphus lotus*
E. Jujube; African Lotus
F. Jujubier de la Berberie
G. Lotusbaum;
    Judendornbeeren
S. Lotusbröstbär
Sp. Azufaifo loto
It. Giuggiolo; Loto
Gr. Tzitzifiá
Gr. Τζιτζιφιά
H. Európai jujubafa
P. Jujuba
T. Hünnap; Çiğde

PART II

THE INDEXES

English Index

Ginger 754
Ginger, Wild 86
Gingko 330
Ginseng 500
Ginseng, Siberian 276
Glasswort 621
Globeflower 332
Globularia, common 332
Goat's Beard 705
Goat's Rue 315
Golden Rain 389
Golden Rod 662
Goldenseal 360
Good King Henry 174
Gooseberry 606
Goosefoot 174
Goosefoot, white 172
Goosegrass 319
Gorse 717
Gotu Kola 361
Goutweed 18
Grape 747a
Grapefruit 199
Grapevine 747
Gravel Root 295
Great Reedmace 716
Greater Plantain 544
Green Hellebore 348
Green Pepper 138
Grindilia 339
Gromwell 414
Ground Elder 18
Ground Ivy 331
Groundnut 68
Groundsel 646
Guaiacum 340
Guar 239
Guarana 509
Guava 583
Guelder Rose 738
Gulfweed 634
Gum Arabic 4
Gum Rockrose 193
Gum Tragacanth 94
Gum, ammoniac 264
Gumbo 353

Gumplant 339
Gypsywort 426

Hackberry 157
Hare's Ear 121
Hart's Tongue Fern 521
Hawthorn 226
Hazelnut 224
Heartease 744
Heather 127
Hedge Garlic 31
Hedge Hyssop 338
Hellebore, black 347
Hellebore, false 17
Hellebore, green 348
Hellebore, white 731
Hemlock 215
Hemp 135
Hemp Agrimony 293
Hempweed 295
Hemp, Canadian 66
Hemp-nettle, common 316
Henbane 362
Henna 400
Herb Paris 505
Herb Robert 327
Herniary 351
Hibiscus 354
Hog's Fennel 515
Hogweed 350
Holly 366
Holly, sea 286
Hollyhock 43
Holy Grass 59
Holy Thistle 204
Honeysuckle 419
Hops 358
Horehound, black 99
Horehound, water 426
Horehound, white 440
Hornbeam 146
Horse balm 211
Horse chestnut 19
Horsemint 461
Horsenettle 657
Horseradish Tree 462

Index Français

Deutscher Index

Gelbwurzel 237
Gelbwurzel, Kanadische 360
Gemüsebanane 466
Germer, weisser 731
Gerste 357
Gewöhnlicher Blutweiderach 429
Gewöhnliche Acker Frauenmantel 26
Gewönliche Haselwurz 86
Gewöhnliche Kugelblume 332
Gewölniches Meertraubel 278
Gewürzkerbel 69
Gewürzstrauch 129
Giftlattich 392
Gingko 330
Ginseng 500
Ginseng, Amazonischer 518
Ginster, Spanischer 665
Glaskraut 504
Glasschmaltz 621
Gnadenkraut 338
Golddistel 145
Goldlack 169
Goldmelisse 460
Goldregen 389
Goldrute, echte 662
Gottesurteilbohne 523
Granatapfel 587
Grau Pappel 562
Grindelkraut 339
Grüne-Minze 453
Guar 239
Guarana 509
Guave 583
Guayac 340
Gummi arabischer 4
Gummitragant 94
Gummizistrose 193
Gundelrebe 331
Gundermann 331
Günsel 24
Gurke 233
Gurkenkraut 53
Guter Heinrich 174

Hafer 97
Haferwurzel 704
Hagrose 608

Hahnenfuss 153
Hainbuche 146
Hanf 135
Hanfhundsgift 66
Hängeweide 638
Harnkraut 175
Haselnuss 224
Haselwurz 86
Hauhechel, dornige 487
Hauswurz 644
Heidelbeere 725
Heidenkraut 127
Heikdorn 299
Heiligenkraut, Graues 632
Heil-Zeist 106
Hennastrauch 400
Herbst-Adonisröschen 17
Herbstfeuerröschen 15
Herbstseidelbast 250
Herbstzeitlose 210
Herkuleskraut 350
Herzgespann 402
Heusamen 546
Hibiskus 354
Himbeere 613
Himmelsleiter 551
Hirschzunge 521
Hirse 501
Hirtentäschel 137
Hohler Lerchensporn 223
Hohlwurzel, lange 75
Hohlzahn 316
Holunder 627
Holzapfel 433
Hopfen 358
Hopfenseide 238
Hornklee, gemeiner 421
Hortensie 359
Huflattich 715
Hundrose 608
Hundsgift 65
Hundspetersilie 20
Hundszunge 245

Immenblatt 449
Immergün, grosses 741
Indianertabak 417

Svenska Index

Índice Español

Espinardo 623
Espino amarillo 356
Espino blanco 226
Espino cerval 599
Espliego 398
Espolon 202
Espuela silvestre 216
Estilos de maíz 753
Estragón 82
Estramonia 252
Estropajo 422
Esula redonda 297
Estepa 193
Eucalipto 290
Eufrasia 298
Eupatoria 295
Eupatorio de agua 293
Evónimo 292

Farfara 513
Fayera 270
Felandrio acuatico 484
Fenicula 306
Fenogreco 708
Filipendula 305
Filipodio 560
Fitolaca 524
Flor de nieve 314
Flor de pasion 507
Flor de primaver 571
Frambuesa negra 612
Frambuesa 613
Freno del diablo 638
Fresa 307
Fresno 309
Fuco vejigoso 311
Fumaria 312

Gagea de los campos 313
Galanga menor 41
Galbano 302
Galega 315
Galeopsis 316
Galio 320
Gallarito 510

Gallocresta 625
Garanza 611
Garbanzo 181
Gariofilea 329
Gatuña 487
Gaulteria 321
Gayomba 665
Gayuba 72
Gelsomina 323
Genciana 325
Geranio malva 511
Geranio silvestre 326
Germandria 695
Gingibre 754
Gingko 330
Ginistra y groto romero 620
Ginseng brazilero 518
Ginseng 500
Girasol 344
Glasto 376
Globularia mayor 332
Golondrina 296
Goma arabica 4
Gorbiza 510
Gordolobo 733
Gordolobollo 571
Gota de sangre 14
Graciola 338
Grama de olor 59
Grama 23
Grama roja 143
Granado 587
Gratabous 159
Grindelia 339
Grosellero negro 604
Grosellero 605
Grosello espinosa 606
Guar 239
Guaraná 509
Guataco 598
Guayabo 583
Guayacan 340
Guayaco 340
Guindal 576
Guindo garrafal 576

Indice Italiano

213

Aristolochia 75
Armeria marittima 77
Arnica 79
Artemisia volgare 83
Artiglio del diavolo 342
Asaro 86
Asclepiade 87
Asparago 88
Asfodelo 91
Asperula odorosa 89
Assafetida 301
Assenzio roano 81
Assenzio selvatico 83
Astragalo vero 93
Atanasia 692
Atriplice 95
Attaccamani 319
Avena 97
Avocato 512
Azadarac 98

Baccaro 86
Bagolaro 157
Ballota 99
Balsamo del Peru 471
Balsamo del Tolu 472
Balsamo di Mecca 214
Balsamo di Palestina 214
Balsamo storace 412
Banana 465
Barancio 107
Barba di becco 705
Barba di San Cristoforo 12
Barba granoturco 753
Barbabietola 105
Barbaforte 205
Barboncino limone 242
Barbone 119
Barbotino 689
Bardana 71
Basilico 483
Beccabunga 735
Bella di undiciore 495
Belladonna 96
Benedetta 328
Benzoino 677

Berbero 104
Berberi 431
Bergamotto 197
Bergamotto 460
Berretta da prete 292
Betel 536
Betonica 106
Betulla 107
Biada 97
Biancospino 226
Billeri 141
Biondella 160
Bisnaga 47
Bistorta 557
Blito 44
Blito 46
Boca di lupe 449
Bocca di cucio 285
Boldo del Cile 517
Borragina 109
Borrana 109
Sesame 648
Shallot 32
Shepherd's Purse 137
Silk Cotton Tree 156
Silver Birch 107
Silver Fir 1
Silverweed 566
Skullcap 640
Bucaneve 314
Bucco 102
Bugula 24
Bursa pastoris 137
Butolo d'acqua 672

Cacao 699
Cacto 643
Caffè 208
Caglio asprello 319
Caglio giallo 320
Cajeput 446
Calamo aromatico 11
Calcatreppolo marittimo 286
Calcatreppolo campestre 285
Calderugia 646
Calendula 125

Greek Transliteration

Ελληνικο Ευρετηριο

Αλμιριά 227
Αλμιρίκι 621
Αλμιρικιά 227
Αλόη 39
Αλόχι 39
Αλπινιά 41
Αλφάλφα 444
Αλχεμίλλα η αρουαία 26
Αλχιμίλλα η κοινή 27
Αμαμηλίς 341
Αμάραντο 346
Αμάραντος 45
Αμμονίακον κόμμι 264
Αμμόχορτα 249
Αμπελόκλιμα 747
Άμπελος 747
Αμπελουρίδα 119
Αμύγδαλον 48
Αναγαλλίς κίτρινη 427
Ανάγκαλις 50
Ανάλατος 162
Ανανάς 51
Ανγκοστούρα 318
Ανδράκλα 565
Άνηθος 53
Ανθέμις η βαφική 58
Ανθόξανθο 59
Ανθύλλις 62
Αντεννάρια 56
Αντίδι 182
Απάπικο φυστίκι 68
Απίγανος 619
Απόκυνον το ανδροσαιμόφυλλον 65
Απόμυνον το κανάβιον 66
Απούρονος 5
Απρονιά 5
Αραβικόν κόμμι 4
Αρακάς 542
Αράλια 69
Αρενάρια 143
Αρενάρια 74
Αρενόπτερις 270
Αριστολόχια 75
Αριστολόχια 76
Αρκουδοστάφυλο 72
Αρμερία 77

Αρμυρίκι 687
Αρνικί 79
Άρον 84
Αρπαγόφυτο 342
Αρραρούτι 439
Αρτεμισία η κοινί 83
Ασαρόν 86
Ασιφαίτιδα 301
Ασκλεπιός 87
Ασκληπιάδα 742
Ασπερούλα 89
Ασπομουριά 463
Ασπρόζακι 22
Ασπρόξυλο 292
Αστεροϊδές 368
Αστήρακας 638
Αστράγαλος 93
Ασφόδελος 91
Ατράφαξις 95
Αυλακόχορτο 735
Αυτί του γαϊδάρου 681
Αφάνα 324
Αφιόνι 503
Αχιλλεία η πταρνιστική 9
Αχιλλεία 8
Αχλάδι 589
Αψιθιά 81

Βακκίνιο οξύκοκκον 726
Βαλεριάνα 728
Βαλεριανέλλα η τοπική 729
Βαλότι 99
Βάλσαμο Μέκκας 214
Βάλσαμο 363
Βαμβάκι 337
Βανίλια 730
Βαπτούσα 100
Βαρίοσμος η βετουλοϊδίς 102
Βασιλικός 483
Βασκαδίρα 691
Βατόμουρο 612
Βατός 612
Βάτος η ιδαία 727
Βαφορίζω 30
Βελανιδιά 592
Βενζόη 677

Magyar Index

Polski Indeks

Türkçe Endeksi

Aslan otu 402
Aslan pençesı 27
Aslanpençesi otu (dağ) 25
Aslankuyruğu otu 402
Asma 747
Aspir 147
At kuyruğı 280
Atyaran 351
At teresi 735
Avokado 512
Avrupa ladini 525
Avşar otu 86
Avustralya mantar ağ. 271
Avcı otu 17
Ay çiç 344
Ayakotu 143
Ayıçileğı 727
Ayıfındığı 412
Ayi gülu 499
Ayı pençesı 5
Ayı rezenesi 458
Ayısarımsağı 37
Ayı üzümü 72
Aynı safa 125
Ayrık otu 23
Ayva ağ. 241
Ayvadana 83
Azadiraht 98
Azak egerı 11
Azaron 86
Azılbend 677

Babunek 443
Bac biber 528
Badem ağ. 48
Bahar karanfil 291
Bahçe kekiği 702
Bahçeteresi 403
Buhurumeryem (siklamen) 240
Bakla 740
Baldıran 215
Baldırıkara 13
Bamya 352
Banotu 362
Bardakotu 362
Barut ağacı 599

Basur otu 595
Batı mazısı 700
Batincan 659
Bayır turpu 205
Bektaşi üzümü 606
Belesen ağ. 214
Ben 462
Benefşe 743
Bere otu 504
Bergamot ağ. 197
Beşparmak otu 567
Beşpat çiçeği 317
Betel 536
Beyaz ballibaba 394
Beyaz diken 226
Beyaz dut 463
Beyaz hardal 111
Beyaz Nilüfer 482
Beyaz turmus 423
Beyaz zamk ağ. 4
Beyaz zambak 407
Beyneb fıdanı 250
Bezelye 542
Biberiye 610
Biberiye (yabani) 401
Biberi nane 451
Binbir delik otu 363
Binbir yaprak 8
Birtür deniz yosunu 311
Bit otu 510
Biyan otu 334
Boldu 517
Boyacı otu 324
Boyacı papatyası 58
Boyalık 320
Bozkırotu 351
Bozotu 440
Boz sırçaotu 504
Böğürtlen çalısı 612
Buğa dikeni 285
Buğday 711
Buğday delicesi 418
Burç 745
Büyük baldıran 215
Büyük boğa dikeni 286
Büyük çiçekli 565

GLOSSARY

English	French	German	Swedish	Spanish	Italian
Water	Eau	Wasser	Vatten	Agua	Acqua
Alcohol	Alcool	Alkohol	Alkohol	Alcohol	Alcole
Tincture	Teinture	Tinktur	Tinktur	Tintura	Tintura
Tisane	Tisane	Kräuter tee	Ört te	Infusión	Tisana
Decoction	Decoction	Deko'kt	Dekokt	Decocción	Decotto/ Decozione
Syrup	Sirop	Sirup	Saft	Jarabe	Sciroppo
Oil	Huile	Öl	Olja	Aciete	Olio
Cream	Crème	Crème	Kräm	Crema	Crema
Ointment	Pommade	Salbe	Salva	Unguento	Unguento
Poultice	Cataplasme	Breiumschlag	Omslag	Cataplasma/ Emplasto	Cataplasma
Compress	Compresse	Kompresse	Kompress	Compresa	Compressa
Herb	Herbe	Kraut	Ört	Hierba	Erba medicinale
Spice	Épice	Gewürz	Krydda	Especia	Spezie
Herbalist	Herboriste	Pflanzen Kenner	Medicinalväxtodlare	Herbalista	Erborista
Fresh	Frais/ Fraîche	Frisch	Färsk	Fresco/Fresca	Fresco/ Fresca
Dry	Sec/Sèche	Trocken	Torr	Seco/Seca	Secco/Secca
Grass	Herbe	Gras	Gräs	Hierba	Erba
Leaf	Feuille	Blatt	Löv	Hoja	Foglia
Flower	Fleur	Blume	Blomma	Flor	Fiore
Tree	Arbre	Baum	Träd	Árbol	Albero
Fruit	Fruit	Frucht	Frukt	Fruta	Frutta
Berry	Baie	Beere	Bär	Baya	Bacca
Bark	Écorce	Rinde/Borke	Bark	Corteza	Scorza
Root	Racine	Wurzel	Rot	Raiz	Radice
Seed	Graine	Same	Frö	Semilla	Semenze
Sap	Sève	Saft	Sav	Savia	Succhio/Linfa
Resin	Résine	Harz	Kåda	Resina	Resina
Honey	Miele	Honig	Honung	Miel	Miele
Salt	Sel	Salz	Salt	Sal	Sale
Sugar	Sucre	Zucker	Socker	AzÚcar	Zucchero

Note: In the Turkish names çiç. = çiçek/çiçeği; ağ. = ağacı.

Greek transliteration	Greek	Hungarian	Polish	Turkish
Neró	Νερό	Visz	Woda	Su
Inópnevma	Οινόπνευμα	Alkohol	Alkohol	Alkol
Vama	Βάma	Tinktúra	Tinktura/Nalewka	Tintür
Rofima	Ροφημα	Raöntes	Herbatazeołowa	Ĭçecek
Eghchima	Εγχυμα	Fözet	Wywar	Demleme
Siropi	Σιρόπι	szörp	Syrop/Ulepek	Şürüp
Ladhi	Λάδι	olaj	Olej	Zeytin yağı
Crema	Κρέμα	Krém	Krem	Krem
Alifi	Αλειφή	Kenöcs/Pomádé	Maść	Sürmek
Katáplasma	Κατάπλασμα	Lenmaglisztes	Oklad/Kataplazm	Yara lapası
Kompressa	Κομπρέσσα	Borogatás	Kompres/Oklad	Kompres
Votano	Βότανο	Gyógy fűvek	Zioło	Çeçek
Bahariko	Μπαχαρικό	Fűszer	Zbior korzenie	Bahar
Votanopolis	Βοτανοπωλητής	Növénygyújtö	Zielarz	Mısırçaşe
Fresko	Φρέσκο	Friss	Świeży	Taze
Xerameno	Ξεραμένο	Szárasz	Suchy	Kuru
Horta	Χόρτα	Fű	Trawa	Ot
Filo	Φύλλο	Levél	Liść	Yaprak
Anthos	Άνθος	Virág	Kwiat	Çiçek
Dhendro	Δέντρο	Fa	Drzewo	Ağaç
Frouta	Φρούτα	Gyümölcs	Owoce	Meyva
Karpos	Καρπός	Bogyó	Jagoda	Dut
Flios	Φλοιός	Kéreg	Kora	Kabuk
Riza	Ρίζα	Gyöker	Korzeń	Kök
Sporos	Σπόρος	Mag	Nasienie	Çekırdek
Himos fitou	Χυμός φυτού	Nedv	Sok	Özsu
Retsini	Ρετσίνι	Gyanta	Żywica	Retsina
Meli	Μελι	Méz	Miód	Bal
Alati	Αλατι	Só	Sól	Tuz
Zakhari	Ζάχαρη	Cukor	Cukier	Şeker